A MEANING-BASED APPROACH TO ART THERAPY

From the Holocaust to Contemporary Practices

Elizabeth Hadara Hlavek

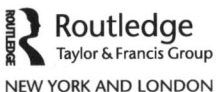

Routledge
Taylor & Francis Group

NEW YORK AND LONDON

Cover image: © Alice Ehrmann Shek (1927–2007). *Untitled.* Terezín, 1943. Property of the Shek family.

First published 2023
by Routledge
605 Third Avenue, New York, NY 10158

and by Routledge
4 Park Square, Milton Park, Abingdon, Oxon, OX14 4RN

Routledge is an imprint of the Taylor & Francis Group, an informa business

Library of Congress Cataloging-in-Publication Data
Names: Hlavek, Elizabeth Hadara, author.
Title: A meaning based approach to art therapy : from the holocaust to contemporary practices / Elizabeth Hadara Hlavek.
Description: New York, NY : Routledge, 2023. | Includes bibliographical references and index. |
Identifiers: LCCN 2022009877 (print) | LCCN 2022009878 (ebook) |
ISBN 9780367750770 (hardback) | ISBN 9780367750763 (paperback) |
ISBN 9781003160885 (ebook)
Subjects: LCSH: Logotherapy. | Art therapy. | Phenomenological psychology. |
Holocaust, Jewish (1939-1945)–Psychological aspects.
Classification: LCC RC489.L6 H53 2023 (print) | LCC RC489.L6 (ebook) |
DDC 616.89/1656–dc23/eng/20220629
LC record available at https://lccn.loc.gov/2022009877
LC ebook record available at https://lccn.loc.gov/2022009878

ISBN: 978-0-367-75077-0 (hbk)
ISBN: 978-0-367-75076-3 (pbk)
ISBN: 978-1-003-16088-5 (ebk)

DOI: 10.4324/9781003160885

Typeset in Baskerville
by KnowledgeWorks Global Ltd.

A MEANING-BASED APPROACH TO ART THERAPY

A Meaning-Based Approach to Art Therapy contextualizes the phenomenon of Holocaust artwork in the field of art therapy and uses this canon of artwork to support the inclusion of logotherapy in art therapy theory and practice.

The author expounds on a study in which she interviewed surviving Holocaust artists about how they were able to create their artworks while in Nazi captivity. Divided into three parts, the book follows the chronological order of her inquiry. It first presents theory, then research, and ends with implications for the practice of art therapy. The research chapters set out the process and results of the author's phenomenological inquiry. They address how art making during the Holocaust allowed captive artists to bear witness, leave a legacy and retain their humanity. In the final part, the author reveals how art therapists can use concepts from her study to support the progress of their clients. She advocates for the application of logotherapy, an existential philosophy that emphasizes finding meaning to facilitate healing and personal growth.

Practicing art therapists and students of art therapy will find this book to be an excellent resource on logotherapy, an updated perspective on existentialism, and a contemporary examination of phenomenology.

Elizabeth Hadara Hlavek, DAT, ATR-BC, LCPAT is an art therapist in private practice in Annapolis, Maryland. She is committed to art therapy advocacy and worked with state legislators to develop the first clinical art therapy license in the state of Maryland. She has served on the Maryland Board of Professional Counselors and Therapists and on the board of directors of the American Art Therapy Association.

"This book traces the beginnings of logotherapy and explores its intersection with art therapy. Dr. Hlavek's work reminds us that amid the unimaginable circumstances of the Holocaust, the arts emerged as a humanizing force. In the face of horrific suffering, artists asserted their ability to respond with courageous creatively. As such, it is a testament to the healing power of art, then and now."

Bruce Moon, PhD, ATR-BC, HLM

"This innovative book brilliantly explores the connection between art and the Holocaust. Interviewing surviving artists, Dr Hlavek explores the creative experience to understand how victims found meaning in suffering and makes an invaluable contribution to Holocaust education, art and art therapy."

Hana Bor, PhD

"In this extraordinary book, Dr. Hlavek brings us with her on a deeply impactful yet ultimately hopeful journey into the meaning of artwork created by Holocaust victims. With crystal-clear writing, Dr. Hlavek presents her extensive scholarship and research into the use of art making in the face of death and horror. She shares how those who made art during captivity in the Holocaust documented both atrocities and kindnesses, upheld a sense of personhood, found purpose and meaning, and ultimately preserved hope for themselves and us all. Dr. Hlavek's perspective spans beyond individual trauma to provide an existential affirmation of existence and what truly defines us as human."

Gioia Chilton, PhD, ATR-BC, LCPAT, CSAC

In memory of my grandfather, Sidney "Buddy" Levin, who never stopped making art.

CONTENTS

FIGURES

CHAPTER 4

CHAPTER 5

CHAPTER 6

CHAPTER 7

CHAPTER 9

CHAPTER 10

TABLES

CHAPTER 7

ACKNOWLEDGMENTS

This book would not be possible without the narrative testimony of Holocaust survivors and second-generation survivors. I wish to extend sincere thanks to Miriam Alon, Samuel Bak, Judy Jacobs, Frederick Terna, Yehuda Bacon, Helga Hošková-Weissová, Yifat and Thomas Geve, Rachel Shek, Ruthi Ofek, and Sue Peyser for their time, engagement, and artwork. I appreciate their willingness to participate in my research and share their stories with me.

Additionally, I would like to thank Kyra Schuster, Eliad Moreh-Rosenberg, Liat Shiber, Anat Bratman-Elhalel, Sima Shachar, Tereza Maizels, Nancy Hartman, and Suzy Snyder for meeting with me, sharing their collections, and helping me obtain images of this valuable work. I am also grateful to USHMM staff at the Shapell Center Reading Room, who helped me locate texts, videos and archives for my research.

Thank you to Alex Vesely Frankl for consulting with me on logotherapy. Our conversations allowed me to take this work further than I could have imagined and I look forward to future studies in Frankl's philosophies.

Thanks to Larry Luxner for hosting me in Tel Aviv and driving me through Israel to see this artwork. Thanks also to Elena Makarova for welcoming me into her home as a colleague and friend.

Thanks to my clients who let me explore my theories in our sessions. I am grateful for the creativity and humanity that they bring into our sessions. Special thanks to those clients who allowed me to include their artwork and stories in this book. And thanks to Kelsey Dugan for her assistance in editing.

I am also grateful to Dr. Bruce Moon for defining existential art therapy and allowing me to blur the boundaries of retirement. Huge thanks also to Dr. David Gussak for his continuous engagement, enthusiasm, and discourse. And thanks to Dr. Emily Nolan and Dr. Lynn Kapitan for their keen eyes and support during my time as a student.

Warmest thanks to the colleagues and friends always in my corner, including Lauren Leone, Amanda Bechtel, Mary Ellen Hluska, Jill Scheibler, Julia Andersen, Cynthia Young, Rachel Schneider, and Colin Holloway. You have each inspired and supported my work and I am grateful our paths have crossed.

Most importantly, I am thankful to my father and on-demand editor, Gerald, who has always prioritized my education and encouraged my artistic and Jewish identity. And of course, thanks to Adam and Scarlett, for the meaning they bring to my life.

INTRODUCTION

This text relies on the phenomenon of Holocaust artwork to support the use of logotherapy in art therapy practices. I use the term *Holocaust artwork* to refer to the artwork that Holocaust victims created while they were imprisoned in the ghettos, concentration camps, and transit camps set up by the Nazis; or while they were in hiding during the Nazi regime.

I first became aware of the extensive range of Holocaust artwork in 2006, around the time I began my graduate studies in art therapy. Through my investigation of this phenomenon, I became familiar with the philosophic perspectives of Viktor Frankl and how he used them as the basis for his development of logotherapy. The concept of logotherapy suggests that individuals have a deep quest to find meaning in their lives. When that search persists in the face of deprivation, it can become a way to counter the despair inherent in misery and suffering. I have found logotherapy to be a valuable philosophy which I can apply toward my own art therapy practice.

The organization of this book reflects how I approached my investigation of Holocaust artwork and its influence on art therapy practices. There are three distinct parts, each of which parallels one of the three phases of my research.

In Part 1, I outline theories in art therapy that relate to the phenomenon of Holocaust art. I then introduce readers to the phenomenon as a whole, and theorize as to why artists retained their inclination to produce artwork during the Holocaust and how their motivation toward that end relates to art therapy practice. Also, I categorize examples of the artwork considered in this discussion according to a range of themes, including portraiture, landscapes, interactions, pre-war scenes, brutality and satire. And finally, I detail situations of communal art making in the ghettos and camps, which resonate with contemporary social justice practices in art therapy.

In Part 2, I have assembled research concerning narrative accounts of art making that occurred at an extreme historical moment, when existence was "provisional without limit" (Frankl, 1973, p. 98). I describe how I came to this study and detail my phenomenological inquiry into the total experience that Holocaust victims had in connection with their art making. The qualitative interviews I conducted with Holocaust survivors and their kin yielded data that I analyzed using Giorgi's (2009) descriptive phenomenological-psychological method for uncovering core aspects of the artists' experiences. Art making, I conclude, provided the artists with comfort and hope, while reinforcing their self-identities. It additionally allowed them to retain their humanity, affirm their existence, connect with others, and serve as witness to the unfathomable atrocities that the Nazis perpetrated.

In the third and final part, I elaborate on Viktor Frankl's construct of logotherapy, while noting how this form of existential thought emphasizes *meaning finding*—a concept that differs from what Western perspectives label as *meaning making*. The difference is subtle, yet critical to understanding this philosophy. Frankl asserted that human beings are meaning seeking. Unlike other living beings, we, as humans, have a unique capacity to find meaning in our lives. Meaning is therefore not something

DOI: 10.4324/9781003160885-1

that is made; rather, it is something to be found. The pursuit of meaning is what makes life worth living.

After describing the emergence of logotherapy and Frankl's philosophy, I then detail case vignettes to illustrate how I have applied my research on the art and artists of the Holocaust toward my own art therapy practice. I connect the research to the logotherapeutic concept of a *spiritual dimension*—the uniquely human aspect of individuals which, according to Frankl (1967), can remain intact despite external counterforces, even in extreme conditions. I also show how I have incorporated a logotherapeutic technique into my clinical work to support the spiritual dimensions of my clients.

I am grateful for having been able to embark on this research and then share the results with the art therapy community. It is my fervent hope that the individuals whom I discuss in these pages are remembered as artists, not just as victims.

Potash and Ho (2011) found that artwork can substitute for the absence of an artist. With that in mind, each viewer of a particular piece of art has the opportunity to discern aspects of the individual artist that may not be recognizable through other forms of communication. I ask readers to please observe the humanity of the artists whom I have referred to in this text. We should envision them as the unique individuals that they are, or were. Each artist had their own blend of expertise and style, which they fueled with passion, resilience, determination, and hope. It is our responsibility to see them for the meaning they found, as opposed to only what they were forced to endure.

REFERENCES

Frankl, V. (1973). *The doctor and the soul. From psychotherapy to logotherapy.* New York, NY: Vintage Books.

Frankl, V. (1959/2006). *Man's search for meaning* (5th ed.) (I. Lasch, trans.). Boston, MA: Beacon Press.

Frankl, V. E. (1966). Self-transcendence as a human phenomenon. *Journal of Humanistic Psychology, 6*(2), 97–106.

Frankl, V. (1967). *Psychotherapy and existentialism: Selected papers on logotherapy.* New York, NY: Simon and Schuster.

Giorgi, A. (2009). *The descriptive phenomenological method in psychology: A modified Husserlian approach.* Pittsburgh, PA: Duquesne University Press

Potash, J. & Ho, R. (2011) Drawing involves caring: fostering relationship building through art therapy for social change, *Art Therapy, 28*(2), 74–81. Doi: 10.1080/07421656.2011.578040

PART 1

THE ART OF THE HOLOCAUST

I begin this text by introducing the reader to theories of both art therapy and the Holocaust art phenomenon, as the two were introduced to me almost simultaneously. In Chapter 1, I identify aspects of art therapy theory that relate to the study of Holocaust artwork and examine two drawings using Catherine Moon's relational esthetics (2001). In Chapter 2, I provide the reader with a historical context of the Holocaust and then discuss the practicalities of Holocaust artwork, including the materials used and the motivations for creating. In Chapter 3, I expound on six thematic categories of Holocaust art which I have established based on my understanding of this artwork as an art therapist. In Chapter 4, I detail communal art making that occurred in Nazi camps and ghettos and relate this to community art therapy practices.

DOI: 10.4324/9781003160885-2

CHAPTER 1

INTEGRATING THE ART OF THE HOLOCAUST
WITH ART THERAPY THEORY

A panel discussion at the 2016 annual conference of the American Art Therapy Association, titled "Art Therapy in the Real World" (Betts, Duncan, Kalmanowitz, Mcguire, & Rosner David, 2016), provided a discourse on the broad application of art therapy pedagogy. The esteemed panelists described the ways that they utilize their art therapy training to meet the needs of people in unconventional therapeutic settings, including refugee camps and military hospitals; and explained how they have applied what they learned in the classroom as graduate students to their work in the "real world." Listening to this panel, I thought of my doctoral research on artwork from the Holocaust and considered how my own approach differed. Rather than apply art therapy theories to nontraditional settings, I sought to learn from a nontherapy setting to inform my art therapy practice. By studying the organic and instinctive process of art making within an extreme situation, I hoped to ascertain what such artists creating during the Holocaust gained and apply these benefits to my art therapy practice.

The atrocities of the Holocaust are widely documented. Survivors, oppressors and liberation troops alike have testified to the sequence of events in 20th century Europe that led to the murder of 6 million Jews and millions of others from marginalized populations. The remnants of Nazi ghettos and concentration camps can be toured today, further corroborating testimonies regarding the horrific conditions. Additional evidence can be found in the body of artwork that was created during the Holocaust. Over 30,000 artworks from such locations across Europe have been documented (Amishai-Maisels, 1993; Blatter & Milton, 1981), though thousands more were made and destroyed, either by the artists or by their captors. That individuals, stripped of their humanity and fearing daily for their lives, were able to make art in such dangerous and degrading conditions is a testament to the strength of creativity.

Awareness of the artworks created by those oppressed during this time of genocide is limited, even among those who lived through the Holocaust. I believe that this body of artwork deserves more attention, as it offers unique insights into the experience of the era. May (1975) explained: "If you wish to understand the psychological and spiritual temper of any historical period, you can do no better than to look long and searchingly at its art" (p. 52). In this vein, art historians and educators have adopted the term *visual culture* to shift the emphasis of artwork from the esthetic to the historical context and call attention to the potential meaning of artwork within a particular time period (Cherry, 2004). Artwork created during the Holocaust by those who were targeted by Nazi persecution is an example of visual culture. The artworks' primary significance is the context in which they were created and the insight they provide into their creators' psychological experience. I believe this artwork is of particular significance to art therapists, as we are trained to appreciate the psychological expression within an esthetic work.

My knowledge of artwork from the Holocaust has guided my practice as an art therapist. From my first introduction to Holocaust artwork, I implicitly felt that the phenomenon connected to art therapy. The idea of creating in the midst

DOI: 10.4324/9781003160885-3

of a genocide seemed to be the ultimate example of the power of art. In the time between my acceptance into an art therapy master's program and the start of classes, I had the opportunity to visit the Terezín memorial. Terezín, which served as a Nazi ghetto from 1941–1945, holds the distinction of being home to a thriving creative community. Visual artists, musicians and actors from Prague and Vienna continued to make art during their internment in the ghetto, in an attempt to retain a sense of humanity and make their hardships worth enduring. Much of the ensuing visual artwork is on display at the Terezín Museum. Seeing these images in person immediately resonated with my interest in art therapy and they remained in my mind as I matriculated through graduate school. I wrote my master's thesis on the concept of art as a form of psychological survival, with a focus on Friedl Dicker-Brandeis and the artists of Terezín. In doing so, I learned more about the artworks created by individuals targeted across Europe and began to draw parallels between different artists in varying settings. Survivor Alfred Kantor's description (1971) of his need to draw remained constant throughout his internment in five separate locations and his experience appeared to be consistent with the testimonials of other survivors. This insight led me to view the idea of art making during the Holocaust as a unique phenomenon of interest. Each testimonial I read had a similar feel: they all suggested a universally experienced benefit to making art while incarcerated.

Gussak (2004)—an art therapist and educator who is well versed on the Holocaust—described his experience of viewing the artwork at Terezín as an awakening, asserting that it may be more informative than any other resources meant to convey the reality of that history. In many ways, the deepened understanding which Gussak gained through viewing this artwork parallels the way in which an art therapist gains a deeper understanding of a client through their artwork. As an art therapist, I can read clients' charts and understand their immediate needs for seeking treatment; but the artwork that they create in our sessions allows me to see another dimension of the individual beyond the symptoms that they present. Artwork made in art therapy sessions evokes the humanness of my clients. Kramer (1998) described art therapy as giving form to experience. When looking at and discussing clients' artwork, I have a concrete depiction of the intangible and subjective experiences they choose to express. I catch a glimpse of their strengths, passions, fears and all the other idiosyncrasies that make them unique. And with this information, I can appreciate and approach them as individuals rather than as an esoteric cluster of symptoms.

I believe that it would not be appropriate to equate the struggles that many contemporary art therapy clients encounter to the years of torture endured by people during the Holocaust. What I posit instead is that art therapists can gain knowledge from the phenomenon of art making that occurred during the Holocaust to inform our theories and practice. Understanding Holocaust artists' drive to create art may help us to better address the fundamental concerns of existence that our clients face. After all, in drawing, painting, sculpting and collaging, Holocaust artists gave a form to unimaginable experiences. The places associated with the Holocaust (e.g., cattle cars functioning as transport, barracks and gas chambers) are among the bleakest environments ever documented in modern history. And yet in that darkness, some found light. Their art gave "soul to a soulless place" (Gussak, 2004, p. 159) and allowed them to retain their humanity.

As I simultaneously studied the art of the Holocaust and advanced my career in art therapy, I noticed other similarities between these two areas of interest: art serving as an outlet for expression in a place where words could not convey the intensity; the sense of autonomy that art making could offer someone under oppression; the importance of creating to maintain a sense of identity and culture when those attributes have been stripped away. Although the context of art making in Nazi camps and ghettos is distinct from that of contemporary art therapy, I believe that the former can inform the latter. Art therapists across the globe work with a spectrum of populations in need of support. Though the specifics of the individuals vary, the need for healing is universal. The current socio-political climate of the United States has contributed to an increase in therapeutic needs. Incidents of racial injustice, the COVID-19 pandemic, the Afghan refugee crisis, income disparity and the rise in antisemitism have exacerbated an existing mental health crisis. The caseload of the contemporary art therapist is filled with individuals contending with the impact of these events, as well as individuals living with psychiatric illnesses. For these reasons, the art of the Holocaust can be an important resource for art therapists working today.

Although the art of the Holocaust has limited representation in art therapy literature, there is research in the field that is of relevance to the topic of Holocaust art. In this chapter, I will expound on existing art therapy theories that have relevance to the topic of Holocaust artwork. In doing so, I hope to bring the phenomenon of Holocaust art closer to an art therapy frame of reference. I will also discuss how the ability of art therapists to synthesize the esthetic and expressive elements of artwork makes us uniquely poised to better comprehend this body of work.

SOCIAL AND POLITICAL VIOLENCE

Over the past decades, art therapists have moved beyond the confines of studio and clinical practices into parts of the world distinguished by social and political violence (Chu, 2010; Kalmanowitz & Ho, 2016; Kalmanowitz & Lloyd, 2005; Sherebrin, 1991; Yedidia & Lipschitz-Elchawi, 2012). In these contexts, art therapy is used not as a clinical practice, but rather to support the individuals whose lives and communities have been interrupted by oppressive forces. Based on their work in war-torn countries, Kalmanowitz and Lloyd (2005) asked how the art therapist can dare suggest art making to one who has endured extreme suffering. The offer of paint or markers can seem insignificant to an individual who has lost everything. Nevertheless, art therapists continue to find their work to be useful to individuals caught in political violence (Kalmanowitz & Ho, 2016; Kalmanowitz & Lloyd, 2005). In her work with survivors of the Rwandan genocide, Chu (2010) found that art therapy transcended cultural barriers and allowed for expression. Although her participants lacked familiarity with most art materials and existed in a culture that did not support self-expression, the art therapy groups were successful in allowing the participants to explore their inner world. Participants gained a sense of autonomy using an array of materials, which countered the depravity and helplessness that characterized their lives (2010).

Kalmanowitz and Lloyd (1999, 2002, 2005) conceptualized the *portable studio* as a construct that serves the process of creating a psychological space for art making in any environment. The portable studio functions for the art therapist as an internalization of the framework of an art therapy session in which participants are safe to be reflective, creative, and able to gain a context for the present, past, and future (Kalmanowitz & Lloyd, 2005). The physicality of the space is insignificant;

what matters is that the space facilitates creativity and ultimately allows participants to "transcend their situation beyond the boundaries of the environment" (Kalmanowitz & Lloyd, 2005, p. 139).

Karcher (2017) brings the discussion of oppression to the United States. He addresses the increase in Americans who have been impacted by political and social oppression, noting the detrimental effect the 2016 election had on marginalized communities within the United States. Karcher suggests that art therapists working with such populations incorporate a social justice framework in order to stay attuned to the specific needs of these communities. He describes how his practice aims to validate clients' experiences and responses to societal oppression, and help them externalize negative messaging and develop a sense of agency. Karcher indicates that art therapy can facilitate a "reconnection with imagination and creativity to make the invisible visible" (p. 126)

Such acts of transcendence and visibility through art occurred within Nazi camps and ghettos. Although their environments were inherently unsafe and insecure, artists creating during the Holocaust were able to internalize their own potential, conceivably reflecting the notion of the portable studio to regain their voices. While hiding in the infirmary at Auschwitz, artist Alfred Kantor (1971) sketched his hometown of Prague, as well as interactions he witnessed across the camp, with the intention to eventually expose "the true nature of this place" (para. 30). In doing so, he arguably was able to integrate his present, past and future, and briefly transcend the limits of Auschwitz. Kantor's art process was beneficial in that it allowed him to hold together what Thompson (2009) described as conflicting realities. Of this experience, he wrote: "I could at least detach myself from what was going on in Auschwitz and was therefore better able to hold together the threads of sanity" (Kantor, 1971, para. 31). Accessing his internalized concept of the studio reinforced Kantor's personal history as well as his sense of drive—aspects that Nabarro (2005) observed can contribute to psychological survival.

TRAUMA TREATMENT

The use of art in the treatment of trauma is well documented in art therapy literature (Appleton, 2001; Gantt & Tinnin, 2007; Levine, 2009; Naff, 2014; Pifalo, 2009; Talwar, 2007; Thompson, 2011; Tripp, 2007). Art therapy is known to be effective in treating post-traumatic stress disorder (PTSD), as it allows an individual to explore their traumatic experience through the use of imagery rather than just words (Gantt & Tinnin, 2007; Pifalo, 2009); and it engages bilateral stimulation (Talwar, 2007), which can support the processing and storage of traumatic experiences in the brain. Art therapy has been used to treat sexual trauma (Backos & Pagon, 1999; Pifalo, 2007, 2009), combat trauma (Campbell, Decker, Kruck & Deaver, 2016) and developmental trauma (Rosen, Pitre & Johnson, 2016), among other sources of PTSD.

I am often met with the assumption that my research on the art of the Holocaust is related to trauma theory. In actuality, I am reluctant to look at the art of the Holocaust through the lens of trauma treatment, as I believe that the victim experience extends beyond our clinical knowledge of trauma. Categorizing this art purely as an example of trauma art dilutes the enormity of the Holocaust. If we relegate the art of the Holocaust to the realm of trauma treatment, we fail to recognize the nuances and implications of art making within a genocide. The artists created work not just in response to a trauma, but during an ongoing traumatic experience in which their entire existence was uncertain. I will elaborate more on my framework for viewing this artwork apart from trauma theory in Chapter 8. That said, it is impossible to completely ignore the abundance of trauma literature when connecting the art of the Holocaust to art therapy. While the artists of the Holocaust were not actively using art to treat the psychological symptoms that manifested as a result of their trauma, there is certainly a connection to theories of how art making can support those suffering from a traumatic experience.

Since the Holocaust experience involved years of marginalization culminating in captivity, Naff's (2014) discussion of art therapy interventions for cumulative trauma is particularly relevant. *Cumulative trauma* refers to the combined impact of multiple traumatic events on an individual in their lifetime. Naff argued that this area needs to be further explored in art therapy, as cumulative trauma is increasingly common. To treat cumulative trauma, Naff recommended an approach organized by preparation, containment, narration and integration. The preparation phase instills hope in the client and invites questions about art therapy. In the containment phase, the client engages in art making to regulate emotions and build a sense of safety. Art can also be used to modulate affect if the discussion of trauma becomes overwhelming (Hass-Cohen & Findlay, 2009). Art is created in the narrative phase to express feelings or memories related to a traumatic event. Creating a narrative of the trauma though art gives the client a sense of control in sharing an experience that rendered them helpless. Lastly, the integration phase involves the client receiving positive regard and support from the art therapist after the sharing of their trauma. The art therapist becomes the witness to their experience and demonstrates that their opinion of the client has not changed after this disclosure.

From his experience as an art therapist working with hospitalized psychiatric patients, Thompson (2009) observed that art can offer "reparation, redemption, integration, and mastery of even the most disturbing traumas" (p. 39). He argued that even near-death experiences can provide opportunities for growth, which people who have been traumatized can recognize in their artwork. Camp and ghetto inmates regularly witnessed death and lacked security in their own ability to survive. These "nadir experiences" (Thompson, 2011, p. 39) appeared to have motivated some of them to create. When exposed to death all around them, some artists became overwhelmed by a need to honor the deceased (Amishai-Maisels, 1993). This is evidenced in the works of Zoran Music, Aldo Carpi, Leon Delarbre and Paul Goyard, who were inmates at different concentration camps. Despite their depictions of emaciated and bruised bodies, these artists also detailed faces and even facial expressions, to remind viewers of the lives that were lost. Music (as cited in Amishai-Maisels, 1993) described the "tragic beauty" that he recognized in the corpses at Dachau, which led him to capture what he imagined as their final breath (p. 52).

Kalmanowitz and Lloyd (2005) contended that "spontaneous art making" (p. 47) as well as formal art therapy encounters can thwart the negative impact of traumatic experiences.

Art making offers those who have experienced trauma a sense of mastery over their situation (Appleton, 2001) while offsetting "feeling shattered and alone" (Shore, 2007, p. 185). In the creative communities of Gurs and Terezín, prisoners were able to come together through their art making, strengthening their connection to each other and ultimately their sense of humanity. Creative self-expression in response to trauma can reaffirm the self (Shore, 2007); afford individuals the ability to address the magnitude of emotions they experience (Jones, 1997); and re-present the traumatic experience to the self (Leclerc, 2011). Shore (2007) asserted that art making allows traumatized individuals to accept and tolerate opposing realities. The concept of meaning making from opposing realities in artwork can be identified in the camp landscape paintings, which include the austere exterior of barracks and barbed-wire fences against the colorful sky and mountains. In a camp or ghetto, traumatized artists could express the horror that they had witnessed and experienced, while also affirming that they were still alive and recognizing that a "glorious existence" (Shen-Dar, 2003, p. 97) might still be possible. By making art in response to tragedy, Holocaust artists were able to accept and reconcile their unbearable reality while resolving to survive.

BIOLOGICAL INSTINCT FOR CREATION

Artwork can be traced back to the cave paintings of Chauvex, France, which are believed to have been created over 30,000 years ago (Janson & Janson, 1997). Ever since, as humans have evolved, we have continued to create art. The fact that art has been produced consistently in societies across the globe suggests that the arts are linked to human behavior and perhaps serve a functional purpose (Kaimal, 2019; Davies, 2012; Dutton, 2010). Davies (2012) saw art as an evolutionary byproduct. Disssanayake (1995) wondered if art making contributed to biological survival—a query she based on the way in which humans pursue, enjoy and value art. Dissanayake believed that since art making has evolved over time, it can be considered a behavior, as it is a trait that has developed with the human race. Explained Dissanayake: "By calling art a behavior, one also suggests that in the evolution of the human species, art-inclined individuals, those who possessed this behavior of art, survived better than those who did not" (1995, p. 35). Perhaps, then, there is a biological basis for the need to create art in the most perilous of times.

Kaimal (2019) builds on the biological need to create with support from neurobiology research, suggesting that art is ingrained in human responses to threat and survival. Given the survival instincts wired in the human brain, as well as our human instinct toward creativity and imagination, Kaimal proposes that art therapy be utilized as an adaptive response to threats. Her model, the Adaptive Response Theory (2019), aims to lessen perceived threats, establish a degree of safety and channel genuine expression.

These theories on art as an evolutionary survival instinct resonate with the phenomenon of Holocaust art. It is often surprising to consider that artists were willing to create in the knowledge that this act would heighten the risk in an already precarious situation. But perhaps the artists innately knew that creating could actually contribute to their survival. Although art making did not guarantee safety for victims, and in some cases led to additional harm, the instinct to make art may have been a survival response. Testimony from some Holocaust artists indicates that art making was an automatic response to the death and danger around them. Jose Fosty, who created almost 500 drawings in Buchenwald, explained: "it's as though you stop thinking, you draw" (as cited in Cognet, 2014). Alexander Bogen also described an instinct to draw while in the Vilnus ghetto and a partisan brigade outside of the ghetto:

> After the war I asked myself, "What have you done? How could you do such a thing and act so instinctively?" Maybe it was a feeling of… let's say, a sense of survival, a subconscious need. I didn't know why I was doing it" (Yad Vashem, n.d).

If art making is a biological behavior linked to survival, perhaps it was employed instinctively in response to threat as a survival function.

The theories presented in this chapter do not encompass the entirety of art therapy paradigms. There are likely additional theoretical frameworks within art therapy literature that further relate to the art of the Holocaust. I share these as examples of how art therapy theory can be supported by what we know of Holocaust art. In the remainder of this chapter, I would like to elaborate on a theoretical dichotomy within the study of Holocaust artwork and relate it to the constructs of product and process in art therapy literature and practice. I will share two pieces of Holocaust artwork to support my argument, before introducing the reader to the breadth of Holocaust artwork in Chapters 2 and 3.

DOCUMENTATION VERSUS ESTHETIC

Art historian Monica Bohm-Duchen posited a dilemma in how to view and appreciate Holocaust artwork. If this body of artwork is viewed exclusively as esthetic, its function as documentation is undermined. If it is looked at solely as historical evidence, the creativity and art process are dismissed. Testimony from artists suggests that their works were motivated by both estheticism and documentation. Zoran Music specifically stated that "my works are absolutely not documents… for an artist it is impossible not to work" (as cited in Sujo, 2001, p. 94). In contrast, Karol Konieczny wrote of his art:

> My drawings ought not to be subjected to scrutiny and aesthetic artistic criticism; an aesthete will not find merit in them for professional analysis. I wish them to be considered a living and shocking document of a world of horror and torment (as cited in Milton & Blatter, 1981, p. 142).

The motivation of each artist may have differed; but in viewing the work decades later, I believe that we have a responsibility to appreciate both aspects, and more. Commenting on the work that she has reviewed, surviving artist Nelly Toll stated that: "In their power and simplicity, this body of art supersedes all aesthetic considerations" (1998, p. xvii).

The dilemma that Bohm-Duchen poses suggests a tension between esthetic and experience. This tension is where I decipher a connection to the field of art therapy. Art therapists often see works created in sessions that are simultaneously a document of experience and esthetically striking. In my clinical practice, I guide my clients to create imagery about their lived experiences to express and explore the related emotion. It is appropriate, then, for art therapists to examine the art of the Holocaust further, as it is not dissimilar to the artwork of our clients. Though the subject matter differs, the overlap of artistic expression and documentation of experience are what we hope to see in our clients' work. Bohm-Duchen concluded her argument by stating: "there are of course no simple solutions to this dilemma – yet the problematic insights this intractable, unforgettable material provides into the relationship between trauma and creativity, and between work of art and historical document remain of crucial importance" (2013, p. 195). I propound that the solution Bohm-Duchen is searching for lies in the hands of art therapists. As professionals trained to view artwork with attention to both its esthetic and documentary qualities, we are well aware of this relationship between trauma and creativity.

PROCESS VERSUS PRODUCT

These differing functions of Holocaust artwork that Bohm-Duchen posits mirror the longstanding tension of process versus product in art therapy literature and practice. *Process* refers to the art-making process that occurs in an art therapy session: the engagement with materials; the tolerance or lack thereof to use certain media; the reluctance or eagerness to make art. *Process* also encompasses the emotional experience that art making yields. Some clients find painting to be soothing and report feeling a sense of calm while maneuvering a brush across paper. Other clients report a distressing experience, like frustration when an image in their mind does not come to fruition as planned, and are constantly erasing and redrawing shapes and lines to match the image they had intended. The process in art therapy is the verb, the action involved in creation. Some art therapists feel that the value in art therapy is found in the unconscious expression and spontaneous art making that comprise process (Kramer, 2000; Dalley, 2008).

Product, on the other hand, refers to the finished art product that can be shared and discussed. The product is the final piece that the client explains and is a tangible, concrete item that sits in the session, almost becoming a third party in the room. I believe that art therapists have historically shied away from a focus on product to distinguish themselves from art educators. The art piece created in an art therapy session is not meant to be assessed or appraised for artistic mastery or conventional beauty, but rather for what it conveys. I regularly remind my clients that I am not going to grade their work, and that I have no expectations for the final product. I look at the art to understand what it means to them and what it suggests to me, based on my knowledge of the client's lived experience.

Kramer (2000) argued that the dichotomy of process versus product is false, as product and process are ultimately one: "When concentration on process results in systematic neglect of or disrespect for its natural culmination – the product – the patient is deprived of both of his goal and of the reward for his labors" (Kramer, 2000, p. 38). Indeed, the product is the result of the process and both are relevant in an art therapy session. The art therapist can see the final product in front of them, but they also witness the process the client encountered in conception. Both are critical pieces of information to the art therapist.

C. Moon's (2001) description of relational esthetics in art therapy further bridges the polarity of esthetics versus documentation. She argued that the traditional definition of the term *esthetics* can limit an artwork to be viewed only by conventional standards of beauty. In this restricted notion, an artwork that achieves esthetic beauty is pleasant to look at, but only on a surface level. It does not challenge, shock or disturb the viewer (Moon, 2001), and therefore does not encompass the full experience of the artist. In this limited perception of esthetic beauty, artwork that is hastily made or not created with appropriate materials is not worthy of being called beautiful. This narrow definition of the esthetics of an artwork can cloud how an individual in an art therapy session views their art. I have worked with clients who minimize the significance of their own artwork due to lack of skill or familiarity with the materials.

In speaking to Holocaust survivors, this same limited view of esthetics also impacted how individuals viewed the art that they or others made while in captivity. Some survivors dismissed the drawings that were made on scraps of paper and cardboard as not real art, since the works were not intended for display or rendered with technical mastery. One surviving artist insisted that her work was insignificant since she just made pictures using sticks in dirt. They could not categorize these frail, sometimes impermanent, crudely drawn images as real art, because they lacked conventional beauty and skill.

Art therapists are trained not to limit beauty to these conventions. We encourage our clients to use art as a form of expression; and oftentimes, what they have to express is not pleasant to look at. C. Moon quoted Levine (1999), who made the point that artwork created in therapy "is often jarring rather than soothing; it is an expression of suffering that strikes the witness to the core; it does not allow for the 'aesthetic distance' which one can take in the face of formally perfected work" (p. 20). Because art therapists are faced with provocative, sometimes disturbing images, C. Moon (2001) proposed expanding the concept of aesthetic beauty to include the range of experiences that our clients wish to express:

> When we are moved to tears by tender expressions of pain, in awe of the courage required or a client to transform internal experiences into tangible form, or witness a client giving artistic expression to something that could be articulated in no other way, we comprehend beauty in forms that deviate from conventional aesthetic standards (p. 137).

Building on C. Moon's argument, I believe that what is beautiful in all artworks is the act of expression: the uniquely human and individualized ability to create a piece of art in a way that only the individual artist can.

C. Moon called for art therapists to consider the impact of relationships in the context of artwork, to include the artist's relationship with themselves, their artwork, their environment and their viewers (2001). She introduced the concept of *relational esthetic*—a term originally coined by art critic Nicholas Bourriard—to the realm of art therapy, which she described as "an aesthetic concerned with the nature of artistic phenomena and aesthetic sensibilities within the context of relationships" (p. 140). In this paradigm, the art therapist's understanding and appreciation of an artwork are contextualized in the artist/client's expressions and life experience.

This notion of relational esthetic can be applied to how we view the art of the Holocaust as a fusion of process and product, a work of esthetic and documentary importance. Many of the works I have viewed are not conventionally beautiful or pleasing; but they do yield what Hillman (1981) described as *aesthesis*, a gasp of sensation and perception. The gasp is a recognition of both beauty and revulsion—a dichotomy that is prevalent in this artwork, as well as the artwork we see in art therapy sessions. Art therapists are trained to view the client and their artwork in a symbiotic relationship. Our knowledge of the client informs our perception of their artwork, and our impression of the artwork informs our understanding of the client.

This positions us to take in the significance of Holocaust artwork. We are able to notice the artist, their experience and the message they are relaying in their artwork.

EXAMPLES

To further illustrate the unity of esthetics and documentarian function that is evident in Holocaust artwork, and demonstrate how they encompass the integration of product and process, I will discuss two particular works. The first is Halina Olomuki's *Six Figures* (Figure 1.1), drawn in captivity in 1943. From a documentarian perspective, the work reflects the mood of the camp. The viewer senses the morose feel of the weak, tired women, cramped together in either a line or a barracks. It is unclear what the subjects are specifically doing, but it is well known that Olomucki regularly drew the women surrounding her in Birkenau. As a document, the drawing makes the viewer aware of the poor conditions and deep sadness that defined camp life.

The need to document these scenes is what defines the artist's process. Olomucki stated that making drawings "became an extraordinary force that carried me to survival" (as cited in Amishai-Maisels, 1993, p. 6). She created these works to show the realities of the camp. According to an article about the Olomucki collection from the Auschwitz Birkenau State Museum, other prisoners begged: "draw us, and thanks to your drawings, the world will learn what happened" (ABSM, 2003).

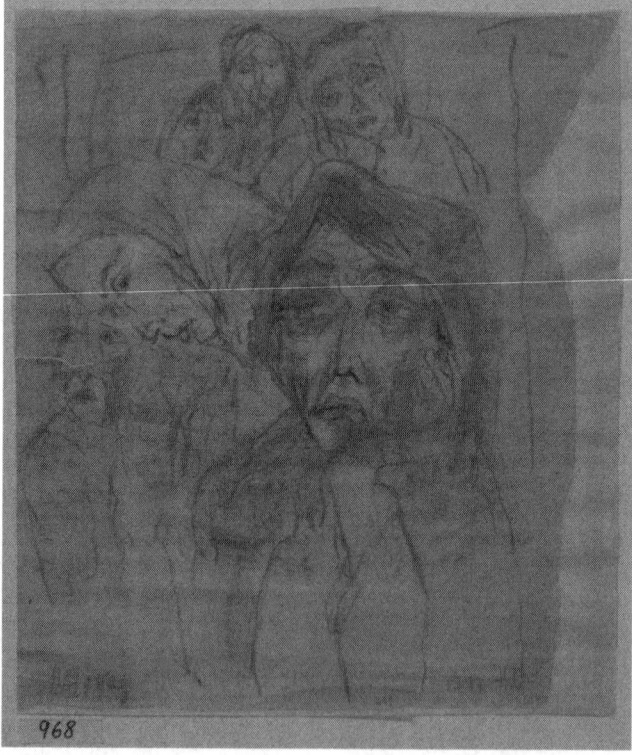

Figure 1.1 Halina Olomicki (1919–2007). *Six Figures.* Auschwitz-Birkenau, 1943. Courtesy of the Ghetto Fighters' House Museum Art Collection, Western Galilee, Israel.

Looking at the product—the drawing itself—the viewer sees a pencil sketch roughly 11.5 × 7.5 inches, on thin paper that was imprecisely torn. Olomucki is clearly a skilled artist, as is evident from her mastery of portraiture as well as spatial reasoning and perspective; but not all of the faces in this drawing are fully formed. The paper has clearly been folded and unfolded, causing permanent wrinkles and creases. This is not a work that meets the standards of conventional artistic beauty and might be viewed by a professional artist as a sketch rather than a great work of art. Still, the drawing is esthetically striking and leads the viewer to the response of *aesthesis* that Hillman described.

This drawing highlights the elements of relational esthetics that C. Moon argued were critical to the art therapist's appreciation of an artwork's esthetic value. There are multiple relationships involved in this drawing that help us understand its significance: the artist to the subjects; the subjects to each other; the artist to the viewer; and the artist and subjects to their environment. In the relationship between Olomucki and her subjects, the artist aims to commemorate the lives of the women around her, who may not survive. She recognizes them as human, even while they have been relegated to death by their captors. Olomucki testified that her subjects had requested she draw them so that they would "be among the living, at least on paper" (Olomucki, as cited in Sujo, 2001, p. 10). In this drawing, Olomucki acknowledges the lives around her. The subjects know they may not live, but they are desperate not to be completely forgotten. Their relationship to Olomucki is one of hope and graciousness for seeing them and acknowledging their existence.

To the viewer, Olomucki shares the realities of Birkenau and the toll it has taken on those held there. She aimed to chronicle the experiences of herself and those around her as proof of the crimes committed against them. Olomicki wants viewers to see the pain that these women bore and to know that this genocidal event occurred. She shows how she and others felt trapped in their environment, confined to a small space, barely able to move or exist.

When considering these relationships that encompass the drawing, the image becomes more significant than a simple sketch. Its documentarian function and esthetic power fuse together to make us understand the enormity of what the drawing represents. It can no longer be viewed exclusively as a document or an esthetic entity, and the process cannot be separated from the product. Together, these elements tell a story of the artist and her subjects, infused with strong emotion and harsh reality.

The second work to illustrate this fusion of process and product, esthetics and documentation, is a sketch by Czech artist Charlotte Buresova, who drew while interned in the Terezín ghetto. *Encounter in the Camp* (Figure 1.2) is drawn in pencil on paper. It shows two figures embracing, with the suggestion of a brick wall and barbed wire behind them. As a document, this image reinforces what we know about gender division in Terezín: women and men were housed separately in the ghetto and rarely had the opportunity to interact. The enforced boundaries of wire and brick indicate that the two figures are being held captive. This image also documents not just a scene from inside the ghetto, but also a rare tender moment that took place within the confines of the ghetto walls. It was important for the artist to witness and document such moments of care and happiness—not for future testimony, but as a comfort to herself. In addition to depicting the horrors of the ghetto, Buresova was known to draw pictures that countered the terror and danger surrounding her (Rosenberg, 2009).

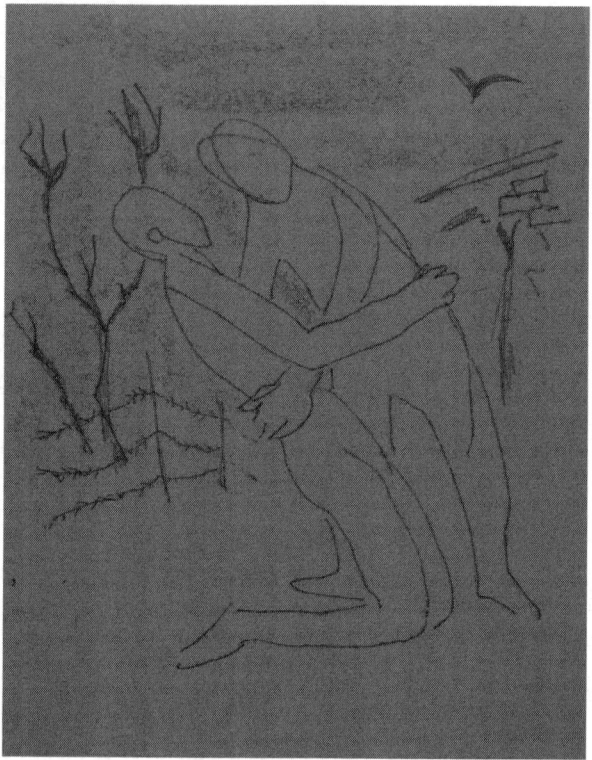

Figure 1.2 Charlotte Buresova (1904–1983). *Encounter in the Camp.* Terezín, 1943–1945. Courtesy of the Ghetto Fighters' House Museum Art Collection, Western Galilee, Israel.

From an esthetic perspective, the drawing is organized and rendered with skill. The figures are placed centrally and background and foreground are established. At first glance, the viewer may not be able to place this drawing in the context of the Holocaust; the embrace between the two figures could have occurred anywhere. It is not until the viewer notices the representations of captivity in the background that the context becomes more obvious. The dark and bare trees give the image a nefarious feel, suggesting that the embrace is taking place in the midst of danger. The flying bird on the right serves as a contrast to the barbed wire and brick wall, reminding the viewer that those inside are stuck.

Regarding the relational esthetics of this drawing, the relationships to consider are those of the artist to the subjects; the subjects to each other; the artist to the viewer; and the artist and subjects to their environment. Buresova's desire to draw this encounter indicates her acknowledgment of a rare moment of beauty between individuals in the ghetto. It is uncertain if she knew the subjects or if she just felt moved by the care evident between them. The relationship between the subjects is also unclear. Their embrace indicates a love or fondness for each other; but without detail, the viewer does not know the precise relationship. We also do not know how long it has been since these figures saw each other. Depending on when this encounter took place, the two figures could be reuniting after a week, a month or years. One figure could be greeting the other after a day of hard labor or upon their return to the ghetto after a death march from Auschwitz. What is clear is that the two were separated and the artist found their reunion worthy of depiction. By drawing this encounter, Buresova tells the viewer that love, care and affection could still be found in the ghetto. These attributes remained alive even in an environment built by hatred and filled with despair.

Through the esthetic qualities of this drawing, Buresova documented a heartfelt scene within the ghetto. In this image, the documentary function is explicated by the esthetic choices of the artist. Each of these two components serves to pronounce the other, placing them in equal significance. Buresova's process and product are also intertwined. Her product is an example of beauty due to her process of deciding to depict beauty wherever possible. In this drawing, each element of esthetic, document, product and process informs our understanding of the others.

Just as there is a unity, rather than a dichotomy, of process and product in art therapy, there is also a unity in the esthetic and documentarian components of Holocaust art. One does not negate the other, as both are necessary to understand and appreciate the artwork and the artist's experience. This body of work exemplifies the powerful use of art in therapy, as it demonstrates the functions of process and product in art making. Robbins (1999) asserted that in an art therapy session, "what is beautiful is what comes alive" (p.177). Applying this quote to the art of the Holocaust, I believe that what comes alive is the human spirit that is observed by the viewer. This desire to create a work of esthetic and documentary value is in itself beautiful, regardless of how impoverished or frail the resulting work may be. I have encountered Holocaust works made on a small scale that appear impoverished. In some, the artist failed to center the image on their surface or rendered the figures inaccurately. An abundance of works depict perverse scenes of brutality or death. And yet, when considering the relationship of the artist to their environment and to the artwork, these images can be perceived as beautiful. The perception of beauty comes from the sense of humanity that is embedded in the work; the bravery that the artist faced in depicting a harrowing scene; their willingness to confront and document the evil around them; their pause to acknowledge and mourn fallen comrades rather than immediately move on.

Returning to Bohm-Duchen's question of whether to acknowledge this art for its function as a historical document or its esthetic value, I reassert that the answer is both. Examining the phenomenon of Holocaust artwork through an art therapy lens serves to unify these components. In the next three chapters, I will elaborate on the phenomenon of Holocaust artwork by presenting the reader with a detailed examination of the topic. As I present historical information, I ask that the reader keep in mind the examples presented in this chapter as a way to consider the art of the Holocaust through an art therapy lens.

REFERENCES

Amishai-Maisels, Z. (1993). *Depiction and interpretation: The influence of the Holocaust on visual arts.* Tarrytown, NY: Pergamon Press.

Appleton, V. (2001) Avenues of hope: art therapy and the resolution of trauma. *Art Therapy, 18*(1), 6–13. doi: 10.1080/07421656.2001.10129454

Backos, A. K. & Pagon, B. E. (1999). Finding a voice: Art therapy with female adolescent sexual abuse survivors. *Art Therapy, 16*(3), 126–132.

Betts, D., Duncan, A., Kalmanowitz, D., Mcguire, M. & Rosner David, I. (July 2016). *Art therapy in the real world.* Plenary presented at the 47th Annual Conference of the American Art Therapy Association, Baltimore, MD.

Blatner, J. & Milton, S. (1981). *Art of the Holocaust.* New York, NY: Routledge.

Bohm-Duchen, M. (2013). Creativity against all odds: Art and internment during World War II. In P. Tame, D. Jeannerod & M. Braganca (eds.). *Mnemosyne and Mars: Artistic and cultural representations of twentieth-century Europe at war.* London, England: Cambridge Scholars, pp. 183–201.

Campbell, M., Decker, K. P., Kruk, K. & Deaver, S. P. (2016) Art therapy and cognitive processing therapy for combat-related ptsd: a randomized controlled trial. *Art Therapy, 33*(4), 169–177. doi: 10.1080/07421656.2016.1226643

Cherry, D. (2004). Art history visual culture. *Art History, 27*(4), 479–493. doi: 10.1111/j.0141-6790.2004.00434.x

Chu, V. (2010) Within the box: cross cultural art therapy with survivors of the Rwanda genocide. *Art Therapy, 27*(1), 4–10. doi 10.1080/07421656.2010.10129563

Cognet, C. (Director/writer/producer). (2014). *Because I was a painter* (Motion Picture). Cinema Guild.

Dalley, T. (ed.). (2008). *Art as therapy: An introduction to the use of art as a therapeutic technique.* London, England: Routledge.

Davies, S. (2012). *The artful species: Aesthetics, art, and evolution.* Oxford, England: OUP.

Dissanayake, E. (1995). *Homo aestheticus: Where art comes from and why.* Seattle, WA: University of Washington Press.

Dutton, D. (2010). *The art instinct: Beauty, pleasure, and human evolution.* New York, NY: Bloomsbury Press.

Gantt, L. & Tinnin, L. W. (2007). Intensive trauma therapy of PTSD and dissociation: An outcome study. *The Arts in Psychotherapy, 34*, 69–80. doi: 10.1016/j.aip.2006.09.007

Gussak, D. (2004). Art made it real: My Terezin musings. *Journal of Cultural Research in Art Education, 22*, 155–161.

Hass-Cohen, N. & Findlay, J. C. (2009). Pain, attachment, and meaning making: Report on an art therapy relational neuroscience assessment protocol. *The Arts in Psychotherapy, 36*(4), 175–184.

Hillman, J. (1981). *The thought of the heart.* Dallas, TX: Spring Publications.

Idinopulos, T. A. (1977). Humanistic education in an inhuman age. *CrossCurrents, 26*(4), 407–415.

Janson, H. W., Janson, A. F. & Marmor, M. (1997). *History of art.* London, England: Thames and Hudson.

Jones, A. (2001). Absurdity and being-in-itself. The third phase of phenomenology: Jean-Paul Sartre and existential psychoanalysis. *Journal of Psychiatric & Mental Health Nursing, 8*(4), 367–372. doi: 10.1046/j.1365-2850.2001.00405.x

Kaimal, G. (2019) Adaptive response theory: an evolutionary framework for clinical research in art therapy. *Art Therapy, 36*(4), 215–219. doi: 10.1080/07421656.2019.1667670

Kalmanowitz, D. & Ho, R. T. (2016). Out of our mind. Art therapy and mindfulness with refugees, political violence and trauma. *The Arts in Psychotherapy, 49*, 57–65. doi: 10.1016/j.aip.2016.05.012

Kalmanowitz, D. & Lloyd, B. (2004). *Art therapy and political violence: With art, without illusion.* New York, NY: Routledge.

Kantor, A. (1971). *The book of Alfred Kantor: An artist's journal of the Holocaust.* New York, NY: McGraw Hill.

Karcher, O. P. (2017) Sociopolitical oppression, trauma, and healing: moving toward a social justice art therapy framework. *Art Therapy, 34*(3), 123–128. doi: 10.1080/07421656.2017.1358024

Kramer, E. (1998). New feature: Art therapists who are artists. *American Journal of Art Therapy*, *36*(4), 100–106.

Kramer, E. (2000). *Art as therapy: Collected papers*. London, England: Jessica Kingsley.

Leclerc, J. (2011). Re-presenting trauma: The witness function in the art of the Holocaust. *Art Therapy*, 28(2), 82–89. doi: 10.1080/07421656.2011.580181

Levine, E. (1999). *Tending the fire: Studies in art, therapy, and creativity*. Toronto: Palmerston Press.

Levine, S. K. (2009). *Trauma, tragedy, therapy: The arts and human suffering*. Philadelphia, PA: Jessica Kingsley Publishers.

May, R. (1975). *The courage to create*. New York, NY: Norton.

Moon, C. H. & Lachman-Chapin, M. (2001). *Studio art therapy: Cultivating the artist identity in the art therapist*. London, England: Jessica Kingsley Publishers.

Nabarro, M. (2005). Feast of colour: creating something out of very little: art making as psycho-social intervention with children of a forgotten war, Sudan.

In D. Kalmanowitz & B. Lloyd, B. (2004). *Art therapy and political violence: With art, without illusion*. New York, NY: Routledge.

Naff, K. (2014). A framework for treating cumulative trauma with art therapy. *Art Therapy*, *31*(2), 79–86. doi:10.1080/07421656.2014.903824

Pifalo, T. (2007). Jogging the cogs: Trauma-focused art therapy and cognitive behavioral therapy with sexually abused children. *Art Therapy*, 24(4), 170–175.

Pifalo, T. (2009). Mapping the maze: An art therapy intervention following disclosure of sexual abuse. *Art Therapy*, *26*(1), 12–18. doi:10.1080/07421656.2009.10129313

Robbins, A. (1999). Chaos and form. *Art Therapy*, *16*(3), 121–125. doi: 10.1080/07421656.1999.10129652

Rosen, M., Pitre, R, & Johnson, D. R. (2016). Developmental transformations art therapy: An embodied, interactional approach. *Art Therapy*, *33*(4), 195–202.

Rosenberg, P. (2001). *Learning about the Holocaust through art*. http://art.holocaust-education.net/

Rosenberg, P. (2002). Mickey Mouse in Gurs: Humour, irony and criticism in works of art produced in the Gurs internment camp. *Rethinking History* 6(3), 273–292. doi: 10.1080/13642520210164508

Rosenberg, P. (2009, March). Art during the Holocaust. *Jewish Women's Archive*. http://jwa.org/encyclopedia/article/art-during-holocaust

Shen-Dar, Y. (2003). Victory for the creative spirit behind barbed wire. In B. Gutterman & N. Morgenstern (eds.). *The Gurs Haggadah: Passover in perdition* (N. Kanner, trans). Jerusalem, Israel: Devora, pp. 95–101.

Sherebrin, H. (1991) Art therapy in a war zone. *Art Therapy*, *8*(2), 30–32. doi: 10.1080/07421656.1991.10758925

Shore, A. (2007). Some personal and clinical thoughts about trauma, art, and world events. In F. Kaplan (ed.), *Art therapy and social action*. Philadelphia, PA: Jessica Kingsley, pp. 175–190.

Sujo, G. (2001). *Legacies of silence: The visual arts and Holocaust memory*. London, England: Philip Wilson Publishers.

Talwar, S. (2007). Accessing traumatic memory through art making: An art therapy trauma protocol (ATTP). *The Arts in Psychotherapy*, *34*, 22–25. doi: 10.1016/j.aip.2006.09.001

Thompson, G. (2009) Artistic sensibility in the studio and gallery model: revisiting process and product. *Art Therapy*, *26*(4), 159–166. doi: 10.1080/07421656.2009.10129609

Toll, N. (1998). *When memory speaks*. Westport, CT: Praeger.

Tripp, T. (2007). A short term therapy approach to processing trauma: art therapy and bilateral stimulation. *Art Therapy*, *24*(4), 176–183. doi: 10.1080/07421656.2007.10129476

Yad Vashem. *The Holocaust in France*. http://www.yadvashem.org/holocaust/france.

Yad Vashem. *The pen and the sword: Jewish artist and partisan Alexander Bogen.* http://www.yad-vashem.org/yv/en/exhibitions/bogen/about.asp.

Yad Vashem. *Interview with Alexander Bogen, survivor and artist.* https://www.yadvashem.org/articles/interviews/alexander-bogen.html.

Yad Vashem. *Interview with Yehuda Bacon, Holocaust survivor and artist.* https://www.yadvashem.org/articles/interviews/yehuda-bacon.html.

Yedidia, T. & Lipschitz-Elchawi, R. (2012) Examining social perceptions between Arab and Jewish children through human figure drawings. *Art Therapy, 29*(3), 104–112. doi: 10.1080/07421656.2012.703052

CHAPTER 2

THE PHENOMENON OF HOLOCAUST ARTWORK

The phrase *Holocaust art* is a broad term encompassing artwork created during, within or in response to the Holocaust. There is an abundance of work from survivors and second-generation survivors created after 1945 which illustrates the use of art making to respond to an incomprehensible experience. These works are a phenomenon of their own and are beyond the scope of this publication. My focus in this text is on the artwork that was created between 1933, when Hitler was elected as chancellor of Germany, and 1945, when the camps and ghettos were liberated. I will use the phrase *Holocaust art* to refer exclusively to artwork made by individuals in ghettos and camp systems or in hiding during the Holocaust. The rare exceptions are artworks that were made immediately after liberation by individuals who remained in ghettos or camps with nowhere to go. These artworks represent a small overlap between Holocaust and post-liberation art. Given that they were made in the exact settings where the artists were held captive, and that their makers remained disoriented and in poor health, they align more closely with art created during the Holocaust than with artwork created later in response. Although many artists who survived the Holocaust continued to draw and paint after liberation in response to their experience, this text focuses on artwork that was made in environments of captivity. Frankl (1973, 1988, 2006) argued that meaning can be found in suffering. I believe that the Holocaust art phenomenon elucidates that, which is why this is the strand of Holocaust art I have chosen to explore.

Holocaust scholars and art historians have documented approximately 30,000 works of art created during captivity (Amishai-Maisels, 1993; Blatter & Milton, 1981), although this number is believed to represent only one-tenth of the total works produced (Bohm-Duchen, 2013). Artifacts from the Holocaust—such as letters, diaries and artworks—are regularly being discovered by museum curators; therefore, any current count of documented artworks is unreliable. Additionally, much of the artwork created in camps or ghettos was lost or destroyed at the end of World War II (WWII). For example, the artist Zoran Music recovered only 35 of his almost 200 drawings after a bombing in the Dachau laboratory where he worked (Costanza, 1982). That artwork was made, and even saved, in the genocide of the Holocaust is a feat that has held my interest for decades. In this chapter, I aim to introduce the reader to the phenomenon of Holocaust artwork by detailing the artistic endeavors that occurred in camps and ghettos. I will answer the questions that are most frequently asked, including: how were works made? What materials were used? How did the artworks survive? However, in order to fully comprehend this phenomenon, the reader must first have a basic understanding of the Holocaust and the terms associated with it that I will use throughout this text. It is important to understand the series of events that progressively disenfranchised German Jews over the course of 12 years, leading to the captivity and murder of European Jews, political prisoners and other marginalized groups. In the following paragraphs, I provide the reader with a historical context of the Holocaust, to make sense of the various locations and environments in which artwork was made across Europe.

DOI: 10.4324/9781003160885-4

HISTORICAL CONTEXT OF THE HOLOCAUST

Between 1933 and 1944, Nazi authorities and their collaborators deported millions of Jews, and others deemed undesirable, from across Europe to ghettos and concentration camp systems, with the goal of total elimination. Those who attempted to oppose the Nazi regime were also arrested and typically deported. Inhabitants of the ghettos and camps lived in overcrowded, unsanitary and overall dehumanizing conditions, surviving on minimal amounts of food and often separated from their families. In some settings, but not all, inmates had their entire bodies shaved and were forced to wear stark uniforms. Their names were taken away and replaced by numbers, either worn on their clothing or tattooed onto their arms. Davidov and Eisikovits (2015) stated that "life in the camps resulted in a reduction of the consciously recognized sphere of identity" (p. 88). All sense of identity and purpose was taken away, to be replaced with suffering, degradation and despair.

The Nazis viewed their victims as less than human and worthy of life only to the extent that they could be of service to Nazi guards or the German war effort. I use the word *victim* to refer to those persecuted by Nazi oppression in order to be consistent with the terminology that most Holocaust scholars use. In the context of Holocaust study and education, the word *victim* has a specific meaning: the Breman Museum of Jewish Heritage defines *victim* as "one who is intended for persecution or death" (n.d.). It is important to define this term in order to fully grasp the cruel and inhumane way Nazi oppressors regarded their captives. They were not intended to survive, and few did.

The United States Holocaust Museum and Memorial (USHMM, 2017) identified the word *Holocaust* as derived from the Greek word for "sacrifice by fire." The museum website defines the *Holocaust* as "the systematic, bureaucratic, state-sponsored persecution and murder of six million Jews by the Nazi regime and its collaborators." Although WWII officially began in 1939 when Germany invaded Poland, the Holocaust is considered to have commenced in 1933, when Adolf Hitler was appointed chancellor of Germany. A leader of the National Socialist (Nazi) party, Hitler was a known anti-Semite and aimed to cleanse Germany of those he deemed racially inferior (Berenbaum & Mais, 2009). While Hitler and the Nazi party specifically targeted the Jewish people, they also segregated other groups regarded as undesirable, such as gypsies, homosexuals, Jehovah's Witnesses, disabled people and any political group that did not support Nazi ideals.

By 1935 the Nazis had enacted and enforced the Nuremberg Race Laws to marginalize German Jews and strip them of all privileges of citizenship. According to the new legislation, Jews could not marry non-Jews; nor could they hold public office, vote or serve in the German army. On November 9–10, 1938, the Nazi party staged an aggressive pogrom against German and Austrian Jews: a total of 267 synagogues in Germany and Austria were set on fire. Jewish businesses and homes were broken into and destroyed. Nazi police seized Jewish citizens in their homes to beat and humiliate them. Known as *Kristallnacht*, or "the Night of Broken Glass," the overnight incident claimed the lives of 36 Jews; approximately 30,000 Jewish men were arrested and sent to German concentration camps, where they were brutalized and degraded (Lowenberg, 1987). Lowenberg noted that in addition to being the most violent pogrom in modern German history, *Kristallnacht* was significant in its intent to ridicule and debase German Jews. He described the organized public humiliation and abuse of Jews across Germany as an "open ritual of degradation and dehuman-ization" (p. 313).

In the months following *Kristallnacht*, the marginalization of German Jews con-tinued. Jewish businesses were boycotted; Jewish children were prohibited from attending public school; and all were humiliated and shunned by friends, neighbors and peers. As Germany escalated its military invasion of neighboring countries, it also attempted to cleanse Europe of the "Jewish problem" (Berenbaum & Mais, 2009). By 1941, Jews in Germany and all occupied territories were forced to wear yellow stars on their clothing, so they could immediately be identified as Jewish. From 1939 to 1944, Nazi authorities displaced or deported millions of Jews and others deemed as inferior from their homes. This systematic subjugation was organized into ghettos and concentration, transit, labor and death camps.

GHETTOS

Approximately 1,000 ghettos were instituted in Germany, Poland and the Soviet Union during WWII (USHMM, 2017). Designed to segregate Jews, the ghettos were initially described as "Jewish residential quarters" (Berenbaum & Mais, 2009, p. 58) and set up in undesirable sections of cities and towns. The first Nazi ghetto was estab-lished in Nisko, Poland in 1939, as an experiment in combining segregated living with forced labor. This ghetto served as a model for others that were formed by 1941. Living conditions in ghettos were unsanitary and filled beyond capacity. Food was rationed and inhabitants were tasked with laborious work for the German war effort. Ghetto barriers were defined by stone walls or barbed wire, and were heavily guarded, ensuring that residents could not escape. The largest ghetto was in Warsaw, Poland, where over 400,000 Jewish residents were confined to an area of less than one and a half square miles (USHMM, 2017). Educational and cultural activities were typically prohibited, although many ghetto residents engaged in underground resistance movements. Beginning in 1941, German authorities began to liquidate ghettos. Residents were either shot on sight or deported to camps.

CAMP SYSTEMS

Beginning in 1933, the Nazis developed a series of concentration camps to detain not just Jews, but any individuals who protested the regime or who were deemed suspicious. These camps were not subject to the German judicial system and there-fore afforded prisoners few rights or dignities. Lowenberg (1987) cited examples of prisoners being denied access to latrines and forced to soil themselves. Over 40,000 camps were developed across Europe during WWII, with the majority in Germany, France, Poland and Austria (Blatter & Milton, 1981). The term *camps* refers to Nazi camp systems that were organized into four categories: concentration camps, transit camps, labor camps and death camps. Although universally inhumane, each type of camp served a different purpose.

The first concentration camp, Dachau, was opened near Munich in 1933. As Nazi power expanded, additional camps were constructed throughout Germany, Austria, and Poland. Concentration camps served as detention centers for political prisoners,

Jews, gypsies, homosexuals, political and war prisoners, and any other categories of people that did not meet the Aryan ideal (USHMM, 2017). Inhabitants of concentration camps typically wore uniforms and lived in overcrowded barracks with limited rations of food and no sense of how long their incarceration would last (Rosenberg, 2009). Many were forced into hard manual labor, without adequate nutrition, rest or hygienic conditions. Guards often abused and humiliated prisoners, and had the authority to murder on whim. In the final years of WWII, some concentration camps became sites for perverse medical experiments that typically resulted in disfigurement or death (USHM, 2017).

Recognizing a need for manpower to support the war effort, Germans set up a series of forced labor camps, known in German as *Arbeitslager*. The conditions in labor camps were also grotesque, as prisoners were exploited for manual labor with little food or rest to sustain them. In some instances, groups of ghetto residents or concentration camp prisoners were marched to labor camp sites to work. According to Yad Vashem, the world Holocaust museum in Jerusalem, labor camps allowed Nazis to reap the benefit of slave labor while also achieving the goal of extermination. This process of "extermination by labor" (Yad Vashem, 2021) meant that labor camp inmates were literally worked to death.

As Germany occupied additional countries, transit camps were set up to hold the deportation of political prisoners, communists and Jews. The majority of these were in France (Rosenberg, 2002), with 26 camps set up in the occupied region and additional camps in the unoccupied Vichy territory (Yad Vashem, 2017). Also known as internment camps, many of the camps in France served as antechambers for concentration and death camps in Eastern Europe (Rosenberg, 2002). After Germany occupied France in 1940 the *Statut de Juif* (Jewish Statute) was published mandating that foreign Jews living in France be arrested and sent to internment camps. By the following spring, French Jews had been stripped of their rights as citizens and deported to camps throughout France. Conditions in these camps were poor: barracks were overcrowded and disease ridden, food was limited and prisoners were deprived of basic dignities. Women and men were frequently separated and denied permission to interact. The largest camp—Gurs, situated near the Spanish border—was built on non-porous soil, meaning that rain could not drain properly and thus prisoners were frequently inundated with mud. Rosenberg (2002) estimated 21,000 individuals were imprisoned in Gurs during its four years of operation. International and French relief organizations attempted to intervene in the French camps. Some succeeded in aiding prisoners with food and warm clothing, and were even able to smuggle children out (Yad Vashem, 2017).

Similar in structure to concentration camps, death camps were developed as an answer to Hitler's Final Solution to the Jewish problem (Berenbaum & Mais, 2009). Death camps, also known as extermination or killing centers (Blatter & Milton, 1981), were designed to annihilate their inhabitants and subject prisoners to humiliation and torture. However, death camps soon incorporated the use of gas chambers in order to kill more efficiently because of the volume of persons being held. Some death camps were located within larger concentration camps. Auschwitz-Birkenau, the largest and deadliest camp, was actually a complex comprising three camps (Blatter & Milton, 1981) and an additional 60 subcamps. Auschwitz I opened in 1940 as a concentration camp, where prisoners were overworked, underfed and abused. Auschwitz II, also known as Birkenau, served as the extermination center, housing four gas chambers and

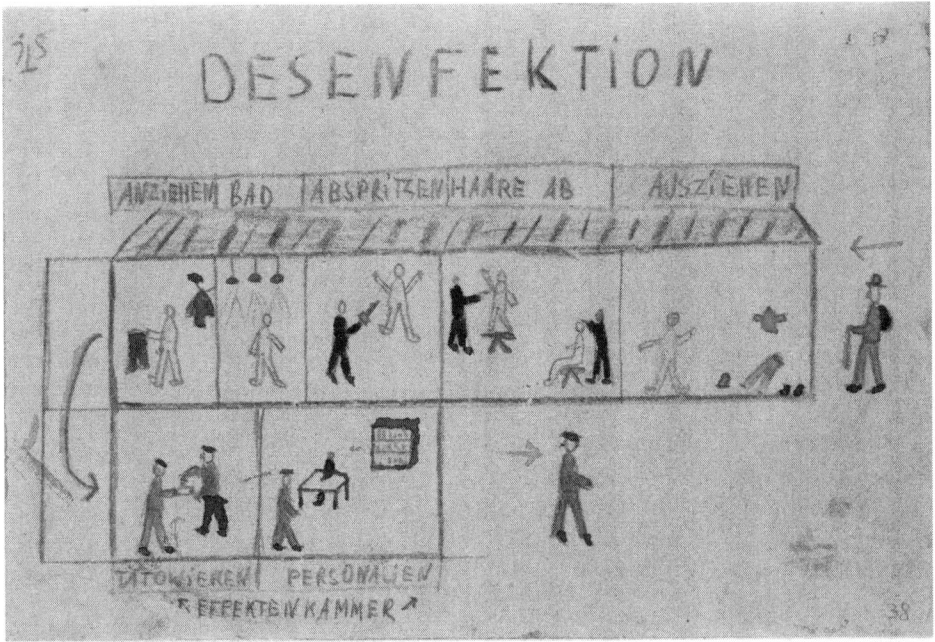

Figure 2.1 Thomas Geve (b. 1929). *Disinfection.* Buchenwald displaced persons camp, 1945. Pencil, colored pencil and watercolor on paper, 10 × 15 cm. Collection of the Yad Vashem Art Museum, Jerusalem. Gift of the artist. Photo © Yad Vashem Art Museum, Jerusalem.

crematoria. The Auschwitz Museum approximates that 1 million murders occurred at Birkenau. Auschwitz III was opened as Monowitz in 1942 as a slave labor camp for men. In his drawing *Disinfection* (Figure 2.1), surviving artist Thomas Geve illustrated the process that he and others went through upon entering Auschwitz.

DEHUMANIZATION AND HUMANITY

In addition to physical torture, Holocaust victims endured constant dehumanization. In a study of 12 autobiographical accounts from victims, Bluhm (1999) noted the frequency with which camp inmates were shamed and humiliated. The dehumanization of inmates was a crucial element in carrying out a mass genocide and occurred daily in every camp and ghetto. In many camps, inmates had their entire bodies shaved as a form of humiliation and personal items confiscated. Upon arrival at Auschwitz, prisoners were sent to *quarantine*—a detention block known for starvation, physical activity, humiliation and violence (Presiado, 2016). This period in quarantine, lasting days to weeks, was designed to obliterate the will of prisoners into fearful compliance. Davidov and Eisikovits (2015) stated that: "life in the camps resulted in a reduction of the consciously recognized sphere of identity" (p. 88). Survivor Levi (1985) recalled: "our manner of living was not very different from that of donkeys and dogs" (p. 13). The inhumane conditions led inmates to become what Holocaust survivors and scholars refer to as the *Muselmann*—a prisoner who has lost all will to live and resigned themselves to death (Costanza, 1982; Davidov & Eisikovits, 2015; Frankl, 2006). Consumed by degradation and despair, the *Muselmann* had no sense of purpose or meaning, and therefore no motivation to survive. Frankl noted from his own experiences that once a prisoner was reduced to a *Muselmann*, they quickly perished. Davidov and Eisikovits (2015) stressed that free will and decision making in the camp environment were essential in avoiding *Muselmann* status.

While survivor accounts of the Holocaust highlight the dehumanizing conditions and treatment that characterized the camps, many—paradoxically—emphasize examples in which humanity persisted. In translating Sara Nomberg-Przytyk's *Auschwitz: True Takes from a Grotesque Land*, Hirsh commented: "what struck me about this manuscript was the author's ability to make the characters in the camp emerge as unique individuals, even against the backdrop of camp depersonalization and imminent extermination" (1985, p. ix). Indeed, Nomberg-Przytyk shared detailed memories of fellow prisoners, offering a glimpse of their humanness. She described her shock when an unknown woman offered her a blanket: "How is this possible… On one side such bestiality, and on the other unselfish love toward another creature" (p. 135). Nomberg-Przytyk also recounted Mala Zimetbaum (drawn by Zofia Stępień-Bator in Figure 2.2)—a vivacious, brazen woman from Poland who attempted to escape the

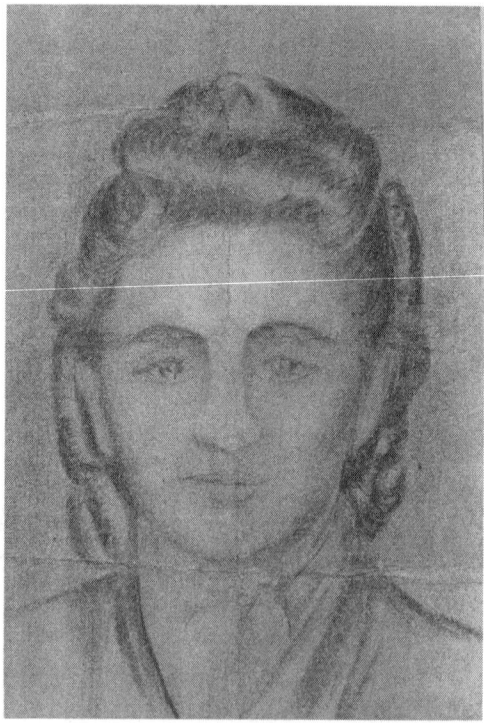

Figure 2.2 by Zofia Stępień-Bator (1920–2019). *Portrait of Mala Zimetbaum made in the camp by her fellow prisoner.* Auschwitz, 1944. Published with permission from the Auschwitz-Birkenau State Museum.

camp with her boyfriend, Edek—referring to the pair as the "Romeo and Juliet" of Auschwitz (1985, p. 102). Mala and her boyfriend were caught and sentenced to death by hanging. Not wanting to die at the hands of the *Schutzstaffel* (SS), Mala notoriously slit her own wrist while her sentence was read, then slapped the SS guard holding her with her bloody hand. Stępień-Bator's glorified portrait of Mala embodies the strength and dignity that she possessed even in her death.

In a similar fashion, Primo Levi (1995) described the relationships and encounters he experienced in the Auschwitz subcamp Monowitz. His anecdotal accounts of comrades and acquaintances are distinguished not by their suffering, but by the characters of these individuals. Levi eloquently paid tribute to those who shared his burden in an attempt to honor their memory and reinforce their humanity. He recalled a surprise encounter with a known criminal incarcerated in Auschwitz, who provided Levi with a favor. "From that day on... I asked myself what humanity was massed behind that symbol" (1995, p. 15). Levi's work demonstrates the victims' ability to evidence humanity in themselves and others—an attribute that their oppressors had attempted to annihilate. He also attributed his survival to his ability to recognize the humanity in his peers: "This attention of mine at that time tuned to the world and to the human beings around me was not only a symptom but also an important factor of spiritual and physical salvation" (Levi, 1995, pp. 10–11).

I share these examples of dehumanization and humanity to illustrate how critical a sense of humanity was to survival, and how rare it was to find. Victims were stripped of human qualities such as compassion, empathy, creativity, imagination, ambition, humor and faith, as well as the ability to identify a sense of meaning in one's life. However, some individuals were able to preserve a sense of humanity throughout the brutality and dehumanizing treatment. Art making is one way in which Holocaust victims were able to maintain their humanity. The artwork of the Holocaust serves as a testament to the uniquely human qualities that were so easy to lose.

THE PHENOMENON OF HOLOCAUST ARTWORK

Despite the abysmal conditions of camps and ghettos, as well as constant dehumanization, some victims resisted through art. Artists of varying ages and nationalities, imprisoned throughout Europe, turned to art making in response to Nazi oppression. Although many artists created their work to document the brutality that occurred, self-preservation was also a significant motive (Moreh-Rosenberg, 2012, 2016). There is limited scholarly exploration of the vast amount of artwork from the Holocaust and no single theory of Holocaust art. Art historian Monica Bohm-Duchen (2013) mentioned that although this body of artwork has been given more attention in twenty-first century art history research, there have been minimal attempts to address the questions of why and how Holocaust artists chose to engage in creative pursuits. Publications from the art museum at Yad Vashem conceptualize the motivation to create as a type of cultural or spiritual resistance (Moreh-Rosenberg, 2012, 2016), which is a sentiment that Holocaust art historians have echoed (Costanza, 1982; Sujo, 2001). However, this position is not universally accepted. Langer (1996) challenged the notion of cultural resistance, given its limitations. He argued that such phrasing confines the artist's experience to something that viewers can tolerate, as an attempt to "redesign hope from the shards of despair" (1996, p.52). The reality,

Langer argued, is that cultural resistance was a meager force against the oppression that victims faced.

Art therapists Elena Makarova (1990, 2001, 2011), Linney Wix (2003, 2009), Josee Leclerc (2011) and David Gussak (2004; 2022) have studied artwork created by victims during the Holocaust. Literature by Marakova and Wix acknowledges pioneering art therapist Edith Kramer, who worked directly with Friedl Dicker-Brandeis in Vienna after Hitler rose to power. Dicker-Brandeis was a Bauhaus-educated artist who was committed to helping traumatized children through art. She and Kramer worked with refugee children in Vienna before Kramer's family fled to the United States. Dicker-Brandeis left a legacy by creating a role for herself as an art teacher in the Terezín ghetto. She began a manuscript, *Art as Therapy with Children*, which perished along with her. Dicker-Brandeis's teachings inspired and informed Kramer's practice and the latter dedicated her 1974 text *Art as Therapy with Children* to her mentor.

Apart from Leclerc and Gussak, few art therapists have explored or even acknowledged the artwork of the Holocaust beyond Dicker-Brandeis or the Terezín ghetto. Leclerc's (2011) scholarship explores the witness function of the drawings made by two female prisoners in the Ravensbrück camp. Gussak has studied the art of the Holocaust based on his own experiences visiting Terezín (2004), as well as through the lens of inmate artwork. Additionally, contemporary art therapists in Israel have discussed the efficacy of art therapy with elderly Holocaust survivors, acknowledging the special considerations taken for this population (Israeli, Regev & Goldner, 2021).

Building on what other art therapists have articulated, in this text I aim to further connect the phenomenon of Holocaust artwork to the theory and practice of art therapy. I draw from literature on the topic of Holocaust art; information disseminated by museums housing the artwork and museum archives; and my own embodied experience viewing such art both in print and in person. Although not created under the guidance of an art therapist or within the parameters of a conventional studio, the artwork of the Holocaust nevertheless can be informative to the contemporary art therapist. This body of work exemplifies the innate creative impulse and its ability to support spiritual growth. Investigation into Holocaust artwork can remind art therapists of the humanistic values upon which the field was founded and provide insight into the depth of what art making can offer to those in need. The examples included here demonstrate how art making can develop and nurture resilience, free will, identity, connectedness and hope. They attest to the power of creativity, which is a deep-seated value of art therapy (Hinz, 2017).

CREATING ARTWORK IN CAMP SYSTEMS AND GHETTOS

Artwork has been documented from multiple ghettos and camp systems that existed during WWII (Blatter & Milton, 1981), spanning from Western transit camps in France to ghettos and labor camps in Eastern Europe. Because art making was so prominent, occurring in a range of locations and spanning genders and age groups, I regard it as a phenomenon. As one might expect, an abundance of the artwork from these locations depicts the brutality of the victims' living conditions; starvation, violence, suffering and death predominated in the camps and ghettos, and were thus common themes in the artwork of those who lived (and died) there (Amishai-Maisels, 1993;

Costanza, 1982). Still, many artists chose to look past reality and convey glimpses of beauty. While drawing in the Terezín ghetto, Charlotte Buresova aimed to "oppose the disaster with beauty" (as cited in Amishai-Maisels, 1993, p. 4). Buresova chose to document the lively cultural life that flourished in the ghetto. Her paintings of dancers and musicians served as a contrast to the suffering that surrounded them (Rosenberg, 2009). Friedl Dicker-Brandeis encouraged her students in Terezín to find and capture beauty whenever possible (Makarova, 2001; Wix, 2009). And Franciszek Jaźwiecki, who is known for his realistic portraits of fellow inmates, also painted images incongruent with his daily life: "I feel a tremendous drive to do my painting, for art that does not know this filth, the misery, and the mean-mindedness that surrounds me" (as cited in APMA-B, p. 468).

Regardless of the subject matter, the significance of this artwork does not lie exclusively in the content, but also in the arduous process of creating it. To fully appreciate these images, one must fully understand the challenges the artists faced. In extermination and concentration camps, artistic pursuits were typically prohibited, so the artists worked secretly, destroying or hiding their work after completion (Bohm-Duchen, 2013). If caught, artists faced severe punishment, such as torture or death (Langer, 1996; Tomić, Milić, Lazić & Marinković, 2019). Surviving artist Alfred Kantor reflected on his drawings, recognizing how dangerous art making was: "On looking back, I realized that taking it upon myself to expose Auschwitz with my drawings could only have come while still very young and capable of being so brazen despite the bleakest of circumstances" (Kantor, 1971, introduction, para 31).

Artists residing in ghettos did not initially face the same severity of repercussions if caught making art. However, their ability to create was limited by a lack of time, supplies and privacy; and by the unpredictable temperaments of their Nazi captors. In an early attempt to keep up the charade that ghettos were designed to safeguard Jews during the war and to avoid potential rebellions, Nazi guards permitted some cultural activities. Examples include musical performances in the Terezín, Warsaw and Lodz ghettos; and art exhibitions in the Vilnius and Lodz ghettos (Costanza, 1982). Over time, however, such activities became prohibited and artists began working clandestinely. Any artwork depicting the realities of ghetto life was viewed as a defiance to the Nazis; and eventually, any artwork not commissioned by Nazis was forbidden. Frederick Terna recalled showing his secret drawings to the established artists in the Terezín technical department, who warned him not to get caught (F. Terna, personal communication, September 5, 2017). Esther Lurie, who sketched during her internment in the Kovno ghetto, recounted the moment that she had to start drawing in hiding:

> Standing in front of the ruins I began to draw. A guard saw me and warned me not to go on. It was clear that I could not continue in the open. I found myself in the attic of an abandoned house. There I completed two sketches without interference... and as the ghetto got emptier and emptier, it was not possible for me to work... I set out to sketch whatever seemed important to me, but it was dangerous to do any sketching in the streets (as cited in Costanza, 1982, p. 97).

Costanza (1982) explained that the Nazis wanted to completely eradicate the Jewish population, including any evidence that they had existed. Artwork by Jews, as well as political prisoners, was evidence of both their existence in the world and the Nazis' crimes. Artwork, and other lasting tributes to anything other than the Third Reich, indicated that individuals who did not fit the Aryan ideal at one point existed.

Works that documented the genocide could ultimately hinder the Nazis' plans. For these reasons, as well as the process of dehumanization, art making was a challenge for artists and much of their artistic activity was done in secret.

MATERIALS

Because much artwork was made clandestinely, obtaining materials to work with was a significant challenge. Some artists were able to access materials through ghetto or camp job assignments (Green, 1978; Kosiec, 1989). Artists in the Terezín design department, for example, were appointed to create propaganda posters for the ghetto. They used the materials they were given for "official" artwork to create their own pieces (Green, 1978; Langer, 1995). Dutch artist Henri Pieck was commissioned to draw portraits of SS guards in Buchenwald and also received materials in his role in the Dutch section of the International Camp Committee, which he used to depict gruesome scenes and conditions in the camp (USHMM, 2021). Artists in the Auschwitz printing and craft workshops were able to access paper and pencils; while others in the carpentry and metal commands used the excess wood and metals (Kosiec, 1989) to make their own artwork. Halina Olomuski painted official signs for guards in Birkenau and saved the materials given to her to make her own pieces (M. Alon, Personal communication, September 25, 2017).

There were artists in ghettos who received art materials through the *Judenraete*, the Jewish councils that governed the ghetto communities. Across Nazi ghettos, the *Judenraete* were tasked with ensuring that German orders and regulations were followed (Trunk, 1972). Ghetto residents themselves, the members of the *Judenraete* struggled with the moral quandaries inherent in their role. In addition to implementing the rules of the ghetto, they were often charged with submitting the names of ghetto residents for transports to camps (USHMM, 2021). In this confusing role, members of the *Judenraete* also had the power to help ghetto inhabitants by providing community services when possible. In some instances, the *Judenraete* encouraged ghetto artists to create artwork. The impetus ranged from documentation (USHMM, 2021) to improving the quality of life in the ghetto (Trunk, 1972). In the Kovno ghetto, artist Esther Lurie was encouraged to document ghetto life for the *Judenrat's* secret archives (USHMM, 2021; Costanza, 1982). Jewish leadership gave her a temporary work release so that she could draw and paint along with Jacob Lifschitz and Josef Schlesinger. The *Judenrat* in the Vilna ghetto also promoted cultural activity, even setting up a gallery to store and display artworks pertaining to Jewish culture (Trunk, 1972).

In camp systems, artists scavenged for suitable materials, using whatever could be found to make their mark, keenly aware that it could be their last. Tiny scraps of paper that today might be easily discarded were treasured and sometimes even offered as gifts or currency between artists. Blatter and Milton (1981) detailed the lengths artists went to obtain materials, citing the use of hair, feathers and straw for paintbrushes. Rust and soot were used as pigments and stored in discarded toothpaste tubes found in the guards' trash (F. Terna, personal communication, September 5, 2017). Ukrainian artist Jacques Gotko used a tire and ink he found in the Compiegne internment camp to create linocut prints (Blatter & Milton, 1981; Moreh-Rosenberg, 2016; Figure 2.3). After being transported to Leibitz, a slave labor camp for women, Esther Lurie drew with woodchips and ink (Costanza, 1982).

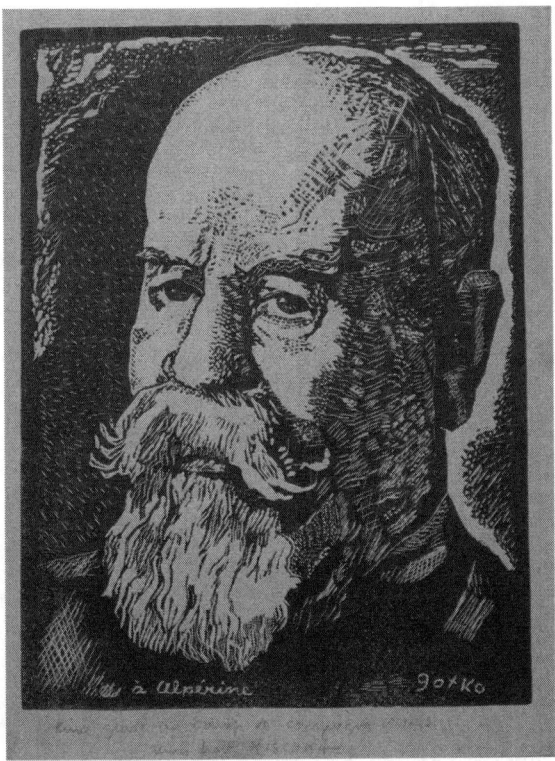

Figure 2.3 Jacques Gotko (1900–1944). *Portrait of A. Alperine.* Royallieu-Compiègne camp, France, 1941–1942. Linocut on paper. Courtesy of the Ghetto Fighters' House Museum Art Collection, Western Galilee, Israel.

Artist testimonies from the Auschwitz collection touch on the found materials that camp artists used. Włodzimierz Siwierski drew on cigarette papers, figuring they would be easier to save (Jaworska, 1975). Władysław Siwek described the way he and other Auschwitz artists made paint:

> First, we made oil paints ourselves. For some time I ground pigment in oil. We 'organised' the pigment in the so-called Bauhof [the area near Auschwitz I where construction materials were stored]. I also mixed paints for the camp museum… The jars and tubes were 'organised' from the Kanada warehouses… Later various methods were resorted to in order to obtain paints. (as cited in Sieradzka, 2019.)

Artworks in camps and ghettos were not limited to two-dimensional pieces. Kosiec (1989) noted that in the Auschwitz complex, artistic endeavors encompassed a range of materials and techniques, including sculptures, bas reliefs and crafts. L'Abbe Jean Daligault—a French priest interned in Hinzert and later Dachau—built sculptures under two inches tall out of plaster of Paris, which he colored with soot, rust, soap and soup (Blatter & Milton, 1981, Figures 2.4 and 2.5). Artists assigned to the carpenters' workshop in Auschwitz made small sculptures out of wood, a material which was in abundance since the camp was constantly expanding (Kupiec, 2006). The Auschwitz Museum holds almost 100 total small sculptures made clandestinely

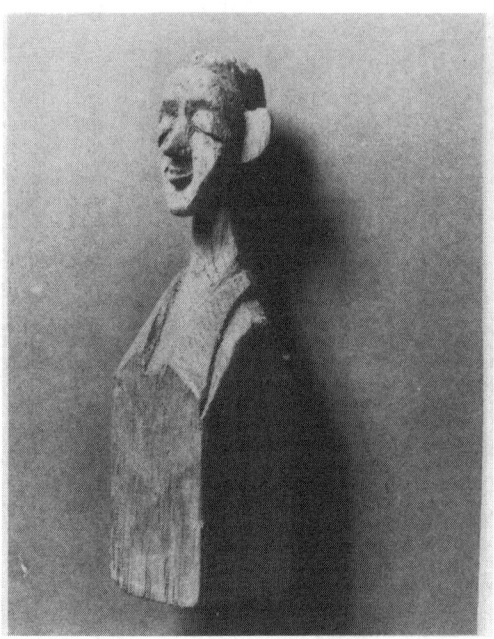

Figure 2.4 L'Abbe Jean Daligault (1899–1945). *Sculpted Face.* Besancon, France, 1943. United States Holocaust Memorial Museum, courtesy of Musée de la Resistance et de la Deportation.

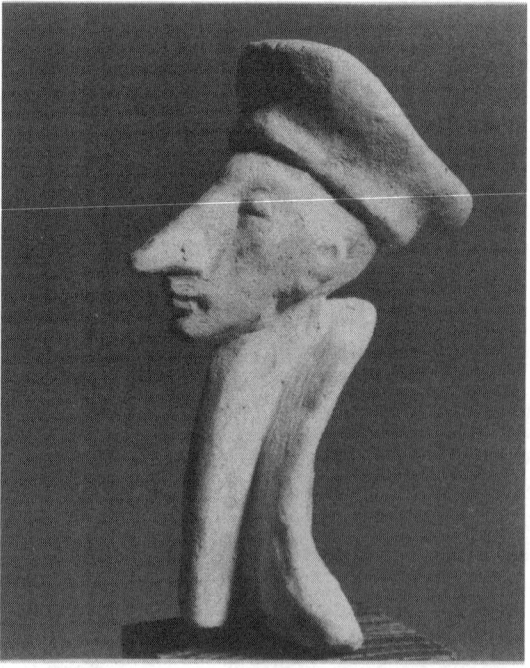

Figure 2.5 L'Abbe Jean Daligault (1899–1945). *Magistrate.* Besancon, France, 1943. United States Holocaust Memorial Museum, courtesy of Musée de la Resistance et de la Deportation.

by prisoners. The miniature size was a necessity in order for artists to keep them concealed.

Polish political prisoner Boleslaw Kupiec carved a wooden statue of the Madonna, which was given to a Catholic priest involved in the underground resistance movement. The statue was hollowed so that a letter could be inserted inside. It read:

> Please help our parents left alone because their six sons have been imprisoned since 16th January 1940. This statue was made by one of them. Address, the Kupiec family, Poronin near Zakopane, No 7 Kasprowicz Street. This message I am entrusting to the hands of our Lady may she keep us ever in Her care (as cited in Dalek & Swiebocka, 1989, p. 2).

Regardless of the despondent environment in which they were forced to live, or perhaps because of it, prisoners worked with conventional materials and found objects in creative, innovative ways, determined to create.

HIDING AND STORING ARTWORK

Since the majority of the artwork discussed in this text was created clandestinely, the problem of hiding and preserving it was especially challenging. The primary means of preserving artwork was hiding it or having it smuggled into the outside world. Artworks were smuggled out of ghettos and camps when captives were moved out on work assignments, which was inherently dangerous. Some artists smuggled their drawings out of Auschwitz on the *Waschetransport* (laundry wagons) by hiding their messages and drawings in the clothing (Costanza, 1982). The goal was to get drawings—especially portraits—to outsiders, in order to convey who was still alive and what was actually occurring behind the gates. On the need to get artworks out of the camp, artist Leon Turalski wrote in a letter to the Auschwitz Museum:

> they were happy to still be alive… that it was him who was in this drawing, that perhaps it will be possible to smuggle his little portrait, his likeness, to the free world, and in this way to notify their near and dear that he is still alive, that he still looks fairly well, that he has survived (as cited in Sieradzka, 2019).

Artists in ghettos entrusted their friends with their artworks when they were sent on transports to concentration camps, as was the case with Alfred Kantor (1971) and Frederick Terna (personal communication, September 5, 2017). When a ghetto artist was assigned a transport to a camp, they typically gave their collection of drawings to a trusted friend or relative for safekeeping. In the Terezín ghetto, Ze'ev Shek kept a collection of resident artworks in a suitcase. When he was transported from the ghetto, he entrusted the suitcase to his future wife, Alice:

> It was a large suitcase, which I hid in a tunnel leading out of the ghetto, close to the barred outer gate. I hoped that it could be found there, even if I did not survive. After the liberation, in May 1945, I retrieved the suitcase from its hiding place and took it with me to Prague in July (as cited in Spenser, 2001, p. 55).

Esther Lurie buried her drawings and paintings in ceramic jars in the grounds of the Kovno ghetto in 1943, though only a small percentage were found after the war. The *Judenrat* hid their collection of commissioned documentary art, including some of Lurie's sketches and watercolors, in wooden crates which were found after Kovno was liberated (USHMM, 2020). Artists in the Terezín design department were able to create a storage place in their wall, which they bricked over to hide (Costanza, 1982).

Artists in camp systems also hid their works in the hope that if they did not survive, their artworks would. Halina Olomuski buried her drawings in barracks in Birkenau and was able to relocate them after liberation (personal communication, September 25, 2017). Jozef Szajna and Franciszek Jaźwiecki were known to hide drawings in the straw under their beds (Costanza, 1982). In a labor camp, Esther Lurie hid her drawings in her clothing (Costanza, 1982).

The concern with how to preserve artwork was intensified by a desire to preserve a piece of oneself. As Alice Shek described, artists could not guarantee their own survival. The artwork was meant to document the atrocities that had occurred, as well as the lives of those who suffered. Because such great importance was placed on these artworks, as in many cases they were all that was left of the victims, artists took great care to ensure their works were safely hidden.

THEORIES ON THE MOTIVATION FOR CREATING ART

As I discussed in Chapter 1, the documentarian function of this body of artwork motivated many artists to create. Sieradzka, a curator at the Auschwitz Museum, commented that while the reasons for art making differed, each was deeply rooted in the artist's camp experience (2019). Artists in camps and ghettos throughout Europe were driven to convey the reality of their imprisonment (Costnaza, 1982). Halina Olomucki (as cited in Costanza, 1982) explained: "My intention was to leave documents about the destruction of my people" (p. 61). The *Judenrat* in the Kosnov ghetto was intent on documenting ghetto life: "We had no camera, but we had a highly skilled artist, Esther Lurie… for the written word was not enough. Without graphic representation the true sorrow of life struggling under the Nazi domination could not be fully documented" (as cited in Costanza, 1982, p. 64). Artists were determined to document the suffering that surrounded them, to ensure that it was seen by others. The hope was that those who perished would not be erased from memory, and that the Nazi crimes would be widely known. Indinopulos (1974) poignantly expounded on the importance of this artwork to future generations: "Unless the artist is listened to we are likely to forget that not the beast but the human is both cause and object of the inhuman" (p. 957).

Little is known about the artist Jozef Richter, other than his desperation to document events. Richter drew on scraps of a Lublin newspaper while on a transport to the Sobibor extermination camp (Cognet, 2013), and possibly in the camp as well. Though small, each of Richter's drawings highlights a scene from the transport, with a description on the back. One drawing shows three men straining to look out of a barricaded window. On the back, Richter wrote in Polish: "Small, high window in a freight car. They ask for water. The guards are watchful. We are on a train on a parallel track. I draw slowly on a newspaper" (Ghetto Fighter's Museum Archives). Another drawing shows a corpse lying on a railroad track. Some show scenes from inside the Sobibor camp. Eighteen of Richter's drawings were found after the war in Chelm, near Sobibor, identified by his signature and style.

Documentation was not the only motive for artists. Some individuals even doubted that their artworks would garner attention from the outside world. Artist

Dinah Gottlibova-Babbit, who was commissioned to draw portraits of Josef Mengele's victims, is quoted as saying: "it never occurred to me to smuggle anything out of Auschwitz. I didn't think anyone cared what happened to us. I just used my ability to draw to save my life" (as cited in Costanza, 1982, p. 51). While many artists created their work to document the inexplicable cruelty that occurred (Milton, 2000), several historians believe that self-preservation was a significant motive (Amishai-Maisels, 1993; Moreh-Rosenberg, 2012, 2016). Bohm-Duchen (2013) argued that the impulse to create art was to "restore some sense of humanity and dignity, even sometimes, a semblance of normality, to the most dehumanizing of environments" (p. 192). Art making is a human act that allowed those targeted by Nazi oppression to define themselves as human. This assertion appears evident in the work of Czech artist Hannah Messinger who, in the Merzdof labor camp in January 1945, stole fabric and thread to make a bra for herself (Figure 2.6) as a means of maintaining personal dignity (Berenbaum & Mais, 2009). She had been incarcerated in three camps over four years, but through this act, she still refused to lose her sense of self-worth.

Holocaust survivor Primo Levi wrote about the loss of self in Auschwitz: "...for he who loses all often easily loses himself" (1961, p. 23). Indeed, the loss of self was a common psychological fate for victims both during and after the Holocaust. Literature, however, indicated that the act of art making during the Holocaust reinforced an identity apart from that of victim or prisoner. While offering a distraction, creativity also served to link the artist to their previous identity (Bohm-Duchen, 2013). In her exploration of works from Ravensbrück, Leclerc (2011) argued that the art-making process provided a way to maintain a pre-war sense of self, as it reminded artists of their past identities. The concept of identity within the setting of the Holocaust extends beyond character, personality and experiences to encompass the artist's sense of humanness. This is demonstrated in the work of Czech artist Alfred Kantor. Kantor was an art student in Prague before being sent to the Terezín ghetto in 1941. Each night in his barracks, he secretly drew the scenes he recalled from that day;

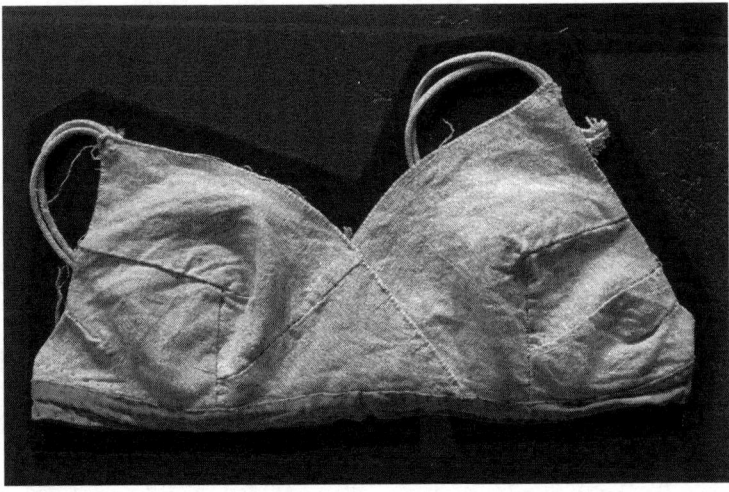

Figure 2.6 Hannah Messinger (1920–). *Stitched Bra.* Merzdorf camp, 1944. Courtesy of the Illinois Holocaust Museum & Education Center. Gift of Hannah Messinger. Photography by Jesus Mejia.

but he destroyed his work immediately for fear of getting caught. Kantor continued this process whenever possible while interned later in Auschwitz, followed by the Schwarzheide labor camp. He explained: "I began to observe everything with an eye towards capturing it on paper" (para 30). He survived a death march from Auschwitz to Terezín and was liberated there in 1945. After liberation, Kantor recreated each drawing from memory. He published his drawings in 1971 as a pictorial memoir titled *The Book of Alfred Kantor.*

Kantor (1971) wrote: "my commitment to drawing came out of a deep instinct of self-preservation" (para. 31). By taking on the role of artist or "observer" (Kantor, 1971; Kramer, 2000), Kantor was able to separate himself from his prisoner identity and envision himself as the man he was prior to deportation. He continued to draw and paint until his death in 2003.

For Lithuanian artist Jacob Lipschitz, who painted clandestinely in the Kovno ghetto, the artistic identity was motivation for survival. In a March 1944 manifesto, Lipschitz wrote:

> Life in the ghetto has broken me even further and I cannot recover. I paint a little, I sketch what you will find here. I live by myself, trying alone to heal myself, as there is no one who can heal my broken spirit. I live with the hope that I will recover and be able to once again serve art (as cited in Moreh-Rosenberg, 2016, p. 192).

Trained at the Vilnius Academy of Art, Lipschitz was an arts educator and illustrator prior to his deportation to the ghetto in 1941. His writing suggests that although he continued to make art while in captivity, he felt depleted and, in his words, broken. The idea of being able to build a career in art once again appeared to give him a sense of hope, even after three years in the ghetto.

In some instances, artwork was made as an offering of thanks. Dalek and Swiebocka (1989) shared the example of a sculpted portrait of Halina Plotnicka, who was heavily involved in an underground resistance movement. In commemoration of the lives she saved, an anonymous artist made a sculpture of her while in Auschwitz. Artist Jan Baras painted an image of Andrezej Harat and his family in appreciation for helping Baras escape Auschwitz. While held in the Neugraben work camp, Marianne Grant drew a caricature of a civilian woman to thank her for sneaking food to Grant. In Chapter 7, I share another example of artwork being made as compensation. Regardless of the artists' individual reasons, Dalek and Swiebocka (1989) argued that underscoring all motivators for making art was an inner need to create.

The artworks from camps and ghettos add a depth to Holocaust education, as they serve as first-hand testimonials from the artists during their captivity; as opposed to survivor testimonials, which were documented post-liberation. The documentary function of this work tells us what happened, while the esthetic elements remind us of the human lives that were lost. If a picture is worth a thousand words, then the art of the Holocaust is worth millions of voices. The examples that I have shared are few in comparison to the breadth of works that were created in camps and ghettos, and by artists in hiding. That artwork was created within a genocide is a testament to the power of, and human need for, art. This concept of art making contributing to a sense of humanity can be applied not just to Holocaust study, but also to art therapy. In concluding this chapter, I would like the reader to consider how the need to document a threatening event or reclaim a lost sense of humanity is related to art therapy practices. Those engaging in art therapy may not be seeking respite from a genocide, but the process of creating artwork within one highlights how impactful art making can be. My hope is that the examples in this text inform the way art therapists practice. Perhaps awareness of this body of art can support the humanistic practices that art therapists employ; or this work can serve as a reminder of how affirmational art making can be. Or maybe the knowledge that art was made in an attempt to feel human within the most dehumanizing of circumstances can bolster the confidence of art therapists, who have historically self-marginalized as less than our mental health peers. Ultimately, this artwork will resonate with the reader in some way, which is why it belongs in art therapy discourse.

REFERENCES

Amishai-Maisels, Z. (1993). *Depiction and interpretation: The influence of the Holocaust on visual arts.* Tarrytown, NY: Pergamon Press.

Berenbaum, M. & Mais, Y. (2009). *Memory and legacy: The Shoah narrative of the Illinois Holocaust Museum.* Lincolnwood, IL: Publications International, Ltd.

Blatner, J. & Milton, S. (1981). *Art of the Holocaust.* New York, NY: Routledge.

Bluhm, H. O. (1999). How did they survive? Mechanisms of defense in Nazi concentration camps. *American Journal of Psychotherapy, 53*(1), 96.

Bohm-Duchen, M. (2013). Creativity against all odds: Art and internment during World War II. In P. Tame, D. Jeannerod & M. Braganca (eds.). *Mnemosyne and Mars: Artistic and cultural representations of twentieth-century Europe at war* (pp. 183–201). London, England: Cambridge Scholars.

Breman Museum (n.d.). Vocabulary of the Holocaust. https://www.thebreman.org/Portals/0/VOCABULARY%20OF%20THE%20HOLOCAUST.pdf.

Cognet, C. (Director/writer/producer). (2014). *Because I was a painter* (Motion Picture). United States: Cinema Guild.

Costanza, M. (1982). *The living witness: Art in the concentration camps and ghettos.* New York, NY: The Free Press.

Dalek, J. & Swiebocka, T. (1989) *Suffering and hope: Artistic creations of the Oświęcim prisoners* (J. Kosiec, trans.). Oświęcim, Poland: Panstwowe Muzeum Auschwitz-Birkenau.

Davidov, J. & Eisikovits, Z. (2015). Free will in total institutions: The case of choice inside Nazi death camps. *Consciousness and Cognition, 34,* 87–97. doi: 10.1016/j.concog.2015.03.018

Frankl, V. (1973). *The doctor and the soul. From psychotherapy to logotherapy.* New York, NY: Vintage Books.

Frankl, V. (1959/2006). *Man's search for meaning* (5th ed.) (I. Lasch, trans.). Boston, MA: Beacon Press.

Frankl, V. E. (1988). *The will to meaning: Foundations and applications of logotherapy.* New York, NY: Meridian

Green, G. (1978). *The artists of Terezin.* New York, NY: Hawthorn Books.

Gussak, D. (2004). Art made it real: My Terezin musings. *Journal of Cultural Research in Art Education, 22,* 155–161.

Gussak, D. (2022). The frenzied dance of art and violence. New York, NY: Oxford University Press.

Hinz, L. D. (2017). The ethics of art therapy: Promoting creativity as a force for positive change. *Art Therapy, 34*(3), 142–145. doi: 10.1080/07421656.2017.1343073

Idinopulos, T. A. (1974). Art and the inhuman: A reflection on the Holocaust. *The Christian Century,* 953.

Israeli, R., Regev, D. & Goldner, L. (2021). The meaning, challenges, and characteristics of art therapy for older Holocaust survivors. *The Arts in Psychotherapy, 74*, 101783.

Jaworska, J. (1975). *Nie wszystek umrę... Twórczość plastyczna Polaków w hitlerowskich więzieniach i obozach koncentracyjnych 1939–1945.* Warsaw, Poland: Książka i Wiedza.

Kantor, A. (1971). *The book of Alfred Kantor: An artist's journal of the Holocaust.* New York, NY: McGraw Hill.

Kramer, E. (2000). *Art as therapy: Collected papers.* London, England: Jessica Kingsley.

Kupiec, J. (2006). Auschwitz w rzeźbie. Ze zbiorów Państwowego Muzeum Auschwitz-Birkenau w Oświęcimiu [Auschwitz in Sculpture: From the Collections of the Auschwitz-Birkenau State Museum in Oświęcim]. Oświęcim, Poland: Państwowe Muzeum Auschwitz-Birkenau.

Lamberti, M. (1995). Making art in the Terezin concentration camp. *New England Review (1990), 17*(4), 104–111.

Langer, L. (1996). *Admitting the Holocaust: Collected essays.* New York, NY: Oxford University Press.

Langer, L. L. (1995). *Art from the ashes: A Holocaust anthology.* New York, NY: Oxford University Press.

Leclerc, J. (2011). Re-presenting trauma: The witness function in the art of the Holocaust. *Art Therapy, 28*(2), 82–89, doi: 10.1080/07421656.2011.580181

Levi, P. (1961). *Survival in Auschwitz* (S. Wolf, trans.). New York, NY: Collier.

Levi, P. (1985). *Moments of reprieve.* New York, NY: Penguin Books.

Loewenberg, P. (1987). The Kristallnacht as a public degradation ritual. *The Leo Baeck Institute Year Book, 32*(1), 309–323.

Makarova, E. (1990). *From Bauhaus to Terezin: Friedl Dicker-Brandeis and her pupils.* Jerusalem, Israel: Holocaust Martyrs' and Heroes' Remembrance Authority, The Art Museum.

Makarova, E. (2001). *Friedl Dicker-Brandeis.* Los Angeles, CA: Tallfellow/Ever Picture Press.

Milton, S. (2000). Culture under duress: art and the Holocaust. In Decoste, F. C. and Schwartz, B. (eds.) *The Holocaust's ghost: writings on art, politics, law and education,* 84–96. Edmonton, AB: University of Alberta Press.

Moreh-Rosenberg, E. (2012). *Last portrait.* http://www.yadvashem.org/yv/en/exhibitions/last_portrait/overview.asp.

Moreh-Rosenberg, E. (2016). *The art from the Holocaust.* Cologne, Germany: Wienand Verlag.

Nomberg-Przytyk, S. (1985). *Auschwitz: True tales from a grotesque land.* Chapel Hill, NC: The University of North Carolina Press.

Presiado, M. (2016). A new perspective on Holocaust art: women's artistic expression of the female Holocaust experience (1939–49). *Holocaust Studies, 22*(4), 417–446. doi: 10.1080/17504902.2016.1201365

Rosenberg, P. (2002). Mickey Mouse in Gurs: Humour, irony and criticism in works of art produced in the Gurs internment camp. *Rethinking History 6*(3), 273–292, doi: 10.1080/13642520210164508

Rosenberg, P. (2009, March). Art during the Holocaust. *Jewish Women's Archive.* http://jwa.org/encyclopedia/article/art-during-holocaus

Sieradzka, A. (2019). *Art at Auschwitz.* http://lekcja.auschwitz.org/en_18_sztuka/ Oświęcim: Państwowe Muzeum Auschwitz-Birkenau/Auschwitz-Birkenau State Museum.

Spenser, T., Tarsi, A. (eds.) (2001). *Art and medicine in Ghetto Theresienstadt: Drawings from the years 1942–1944* [exhibition catalogue].

Sujo, G. (2001). *Legacies of silence: The visual arts and Holocaust memory.* London, England: Philip Wilson Publishers.

Tomić, I., Milić, V., Lazić, D. and Marinković, S. (2019). Psychological survival in Banjica concentration camp due to inmate creativity. A recommendation to future victims. *Austin Anthropology, 3*(2), 1008.

Trunk, I. (1972). *Judenrat: The Jewish Councils in Eastern Europe under Nazi Occupation*, New York, NY: The MacMillan Company.

United States Holocaust Memorial Museum. *Introduction to the Holocaust*. Holocaust Encyclopedia. www.ushmm.org/wlc/en/article.php?ModuleId=10005143.

United States Holocaust Memorial Museum (2020). *Esther Lurie*, adapted from United States Holocaust Memorial Museum, and United States Holocaust Memorial Council (1997). *Hidden history of the Kovno Ghetto*. Boston, MA: Little, Brown and Co., pp. 168–171.

Wix, L. (2003). Art in the construction of self: Three women and their ways in art, therapy and education. *Dissertation Abstracts International, 64*(02), 245. (UMI No. 3081230)

Wix, L. (2009). Aesthetic empathy in teaching art to children: The work of Friedl Dicker-Brandeis in Terezin. *Art Therapy, 26*(4), 152–158. doi: 10.1080/07421656.2009.10129612

Yad Vashem. *The Holocaust in France*. http://www.yadvashem.org/holocaust/france.

Yad Vashem. *The pen and the sword: Jewish artist and partisan Alexander Bogen*. http://www.yadvashem.org/yv/en/exhibitions/bogen/about.asp.

CHAPTER 3

CATEGORIZING THE ART OF THE HOLOCAUST

As I explained in the previous chapter, *Holocaust art* is an umbrella term used to describe artworks created during, and in response to, the Holocaust, which vary by medium, style and the experiences of each artist. Because the term *Holocaust art* casts a wide net, it is necessary when reflecting on their impact and lessons to curate these works into categories which present them in a way that is informative, accessible and approachable. Doing so allows us to identify themes across pieces and view the Holocaust not just through its statistics or graphic imagery, but through the emotions and experiences of its victims.

Looking at the collection of artworks housed at the Auschwitz Museum, Dalek and Swiebocka (1989) asserted that Holocaust art cannot be examined exclusively by artistic criteria and that any classification in that vein is artificial. They recognized, though, that presenting the art in a system of order is necessary for readers who are unfamiliar with these works. The images and history behind them are already so disorienting that classifying them provides a degree of relief to the viewer. It is useful, then, to organize the works in a way that makes them easier to navigate, instead of inundating the viewer with a barrage of haunting images.

To this end, the art of the Holocaust has been organized in various ways in literature. Milton (2000) identified five categories in which to sort Holocaust artworks: portraits; landscapes and still life; documentary art; caricatures; and abstract art. These categories seem to be distinguished by esthetic content. The 2016 exhibit *Art from the Holocaust,* curated by the Yad Vashem art department and displayed at the German Historical Museum in Berlin, consisted of 100 works organized into the categories of reality; portraits; and transcendence. The intention behind that system of categorization was to emphasize the voice of the artist. Explained curator Moreh-Rosenberg: "the portraits constitute a sort of synthesis in this dialect combining the confrontation with reality and the search for spiritual refuge" (2016, p. 39).

Other curators and scholars have chosen to organize artworks by the camp or ghetto in which they were created (Sujo, 2001); geographical region (Blatner & Milton, 1981); artist (Benvenuti, 2016; Dalek & Swiebocka, 1989); or chronologically. Israeli scholar Mor Presiado has focused her research on female Holocaust artwork, finding that this gives insight into the specifically female Holocaust experience. Presidao organized female Holocaust artwork into themes of household work; crafts; motherhood; mutual assistance; loss of femininity; and sexual violence (2016). Such categories are unique to the female experience in Nazi captivity and the nuances of Presiado's distinction highlight the additional challenges of female inmates. Some collections of Holocaust artwork are also organized by artist; as was a series of paintings by German artist Charlotte Salomon. While in hiding in France from 1940–1943, Salomon painted 1,325 pieces in gouache. She compiled 800 of them into a work titled *Life? Or Theater?* (*Leben? Oder Theater?* in German) which was found in France after the artist perished in Auschwitz (Steinberg & Bohm-Duchen, 2006). Salomon's artwork was inspired both by the political oppression she experienced that culminated in her hiding, and by her own family history of suicide (Felstiner, 1999). The paintings

DOI: 10.4324/9781003160885-5

are distinct from other Holocaust works in their abundance, content and cohesion; and therefore are most appropriately organized as the Charlotte Salomon collection. They share elements with other pieces of Holocaust artwork but make most sense as organized in their own distinct category. This presents Salomon's story in a way that maximizes the impact of the art and serves as a reminder to look at the Holocaust through the eyes of the affected individual—in this case, Salomon.

Based on my reviews of existing texts on artwork from the Holocaust, as well as in-person viewings of collections and conversations with curators and surviving artists, I have classified Holocaust art into six categories—portraits; landscapes; depictions of brutality; interpersonal interactions; scenes of life prior to the war; and satire—with some pieces overlapping multiple categories. Since I am viewing the art of the Holocaust as a phenomenon, I did not use geographic constraints to organize the work. Milton (2000) found that her categories of artwork were consistent across geographical boundaries, meaning that artworks from camps and ghettos across Europe all fit into one of the five categories, without distinction between locations. I also found that this artwork was more easily distinguished by content and truly never considered categorizing it by region.

My categories—based primarily on thematic content—differ slightly from Milton's, as I am looking at the artworks from my perspective as an art therapist with the goal of presenting them in a manner that makes them more approachable to those unfamiliar with Holocaust study, and that encourages a consideration of the artists' motivation. To this end, I distinguished these categories by esthetic content, while also considering the impetus behind making such works. What psychological relief did the artist attain from such creations? What messages were they attempting to convey? What did they intend future viewers to take away from their art? Bringing my attention to the visual content and potential motivators for making these artworks allows me to see them as more than just provocative imagery. Taking this approach is a daunting task given the intensity of the works, both in content and in what we know about their creation. It is easy for the viewer to get lost and overwhelmed by the sheer emotion these images evoke, because imagery can conjure a visceral response and imagery representing the Holocaust does so exponentially.

Placing these works in categories more granular than just Holocaust artwork helps to humanize the victim artists by attempting to understand their process in creating. This organization of artworks may resonate with art therapists who find that the response to violence should be focused less on shock and destruction and more on recognizing how individuals survived, and continue to survive, such hardships (Kalmanowitz & Lloyd, 2005). The fostering of humanity through art is the goal in many art therapy settings today. Therefore, the study of Holocaust artists, their works and their motivations for creating offers important evidence to support art therapy practice. In the following paragraphs, I share my examination of these categories to offer insight into why artists may have created and to further readers' understanding of the realities these artists faced in Nazi camps.

PORTRAITURE

The creation of portraits was especially common in camps and ghettos throughout Europe. In fact, portraits comprised one-quarter of all paintings and drawings estimated to have been produced by Holocaust artists during WWII (Milton, 2000;

Rosenberg, 2009). Portraits were often drawn at the request of fellow inmates in anticipation of death and their desire to document what was left of their lives. In detailing individuals' faces, the artist "gave [them] back [their] soul—the very quality the Nazis sought to eliminate" (Moreh-Rosenberg, 2012, para. 1).

Portraiture offered a sense of permanency and allowed those targeted for death to remain "among the living, at least on paper" (Olomucki, as cited in Sujo, 2001, p. 10). This sharply contrasted with the Nazis' view of their captives as insignificant, and with the fragility of camp and ghetto inmates' being (Amishai-Maisels, 1993; Rosenberg, 2009). Many examples of portraits drawn during the Holocaust include the artist's name, the subject's name, the location and the date. These inclusions were risky not only because they identified those who were participating in a prohibited activity, but also because they concretely put both the artist and the subject in a place in time, affirming their existence (Leclerc, 2011). Rosenberg (2009) explained that portraiture offered proof of existence to both artist and subject at a critical time when that existence was fragile. Portraiture also encouraged camaraderie between inmates through engagement, recognition and witnessing of another being, which affirmed a sense of humanity. Engagement between artist and subject created a bond and bi-directional witnessing (Leclerc, 2011) that was crucial for their mutual self-construction.

Portraits captured subjects' particular qualities and depicted them with dignity (Bohm-Duchen, 2013). The individuality and likeness of the subject are key features in the work of Polish artist Franciszek Jazwiecki, who drew portraits of over 100 fellow inmates at Auschwitz, Gross-Rosen, Sachsenhausen and Buchenwald, and kept most of his drawings hidden in his clothing and bed (Figure 3.1). On his motivation to draw, Jazwiecki (as cited in Stiftung Neue Synagoge Berlin, 2005) stated:

> I drew portraits in the camp as a way of finding a short-lived happiness and first and foremost, as a way of forgetting. These pictures I drew in secret helped me forget, they drew me into another world, the world of my art. I was aware that drawing was punished with death and it was not that I was brave, more that I simply ignored the risk, because I could not resist creating my own world. (para 8)

During a routine inspection in his Auschwitz barrack, SS guards discovered Jaźwiecki's hidden drawings and sentenced him to three months in the penal work squad. Despite enduring these severe consequences, Jaźwiecki began drawing again after completing his punishment. He is quoted as writing in his diary: "Every time my work was taken from me I was in despair, but then the greater was my effort and stronger the will to start another picture" (as cited in Dalek & Swiebocka, 1989, p. 3).

Curators at the Auschwitz Birkenau State Museum, which holds 11 of Jaźwiecki's portraits, observed that the only change in his post-punishment portraits is the absence of the sitter's name and prisoner number—likely an attempt to keep the sitter anonymous and therefore safe. Jaźwiecki included the names and numbers of his sitters again after being transferred to the Buchenwald camp, where he continued to draw portraits. The museum's art collection website reads:

> The surviving portraits of inmates are some of the most moving works created in the camps. They radiate with uncommon expression, realism, and power of communication, precisely rendering the internal states of those portrayed. His drawings present specific people, victims of German concentration camps. Confronted with the photographs from before their incarceration or from the day of registration at the camp, they depict the significant physical and psychological change in the inmates portrayed.

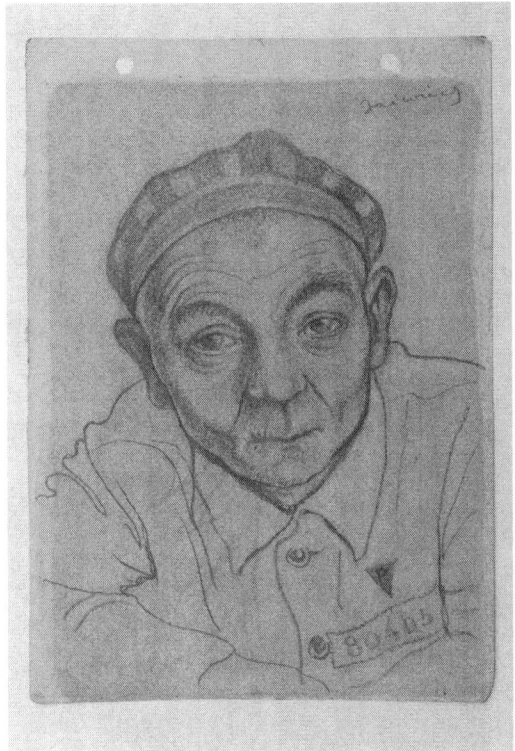

Figure 3.1 Franciszek Jaźwiecki (1900–1946). *A Portrait of Piotr Kajzer.* Buchenwald, 1944. Published with permission from the Auschwitz-Birkenau State Museum.

While Jaźwiecki rendered his portraits in painful detail, artist Zofia Stępień drew idealized portraits of women in the Birkenau camp (Figure 3.2). She attempted to flatter her subjects by giving them long, styled hair and makeup, as if the portraits were made anywhere but Birkenau. After liberation, she wrote:

> I saw their huge, hungry, black eyes and emaciated bodies… Nearly all the women had ulcers, boils, and wounds leaking pus… I tried to make them more beautiful somehow… Everything was so ugly, grey, sad and dirty that I wanted to introduce a little beauty into my drawings' (as cited in Kosiec, 1989, p. 5).

Stępień's act of beautifying the other women highlights the respect and care she had for them. She was able to view them as women worthy of dignity, despite the undignified circumstances in which they lived.

Portraits were also commissioned by prisoners to send to loved ones outside of the camp, in an attempt to prove that they were alive. Ludwik Chrobok, an inmate of an Auschwitz sub-camp, recalled asking a known artist to make a portrait of him:

> He promised to do it. Unfortunately, at the first attempt we were caught by the Block-führer. It was only on the second occasion that we succeeded, and Markiel made a portrait of me on a 10 × 14.5cm sheet. I sent it to my wife through a miner called Witosek (APMA-B, n.d.).

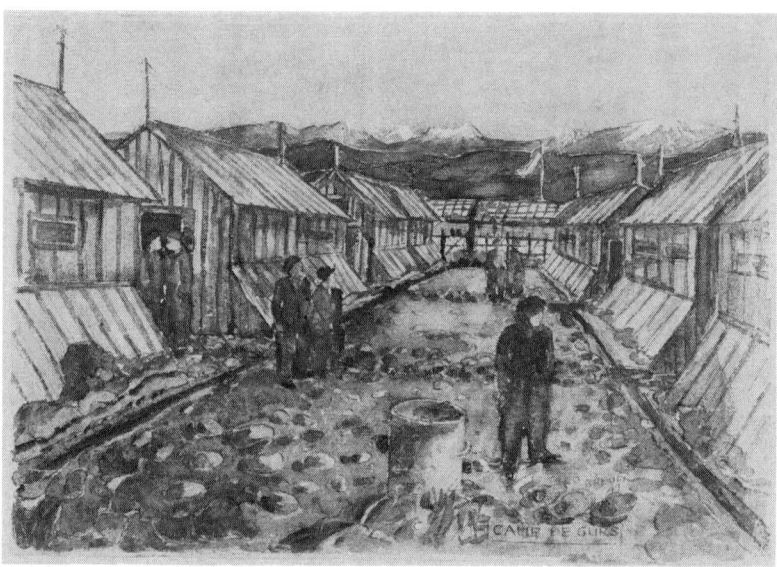

Figure 3.2 Leo Breuer (1893–1975). *Path between the Barracks.* Gurs camp, France, 1941. Watercolor on paper 22 × 30.2 cm. Collection of the Yad Vashem Art Museum, Jerusalem. Gift of Ms. Gita Lehman, Israel. Photo © Yad Vashem Art Museum, Jerusalem.

This example shows the triumph of the need for a portrait to be taken out of the camp over the fear of getting caught. Another Auschwitz survivor, Stanisław Sewera, had his portrait drawn by fellow inmate David Friedmann, who had previously worked as a professional artist. Sewera gave the portrait to a civilian employed at a work camp, who took it to his mother (Sieradzka, 2019.). Polish painter Stanislaw Gutkiewicz painted portraits of Czech prisoners from the Falcon transport, complete with their full names and addresses, in the hope that the portraits could be given to their families in the event that they did not survive (Dalek & Swiebocka, 1989). Kosiac described the motivation for portraits created for others outside of the camps: "…it gave expression to the deepest longings of the people behind the wire – the desire to remind those you loved of your face, the wish to have the image of a person you had lost" (1989, p. 3).

In addition to portraits of comrades, self-portraits were common. Jaźwiecki drew at least one self-portrait during his captivity (Sieradzka, 2019.). Terezín artist Bedrich Fritta, known for documenting the realities of ghetto life, drew a portrait of himself as a laborer. Fritta did not work as a laborer in the Terezín ghetto, though the image of a laborer was a symbol of power and freedom in political art from that period. Moreh-Rosenberg (2016) noted the contradiction of the powerful symbol of a laborer against the hollow and wrenched face Fritta gave himself.

German artist Felix Nussbaum painted multiple self-portraits while in the St. Cyprene transit camp and later in hiding after he escaped the camp (Sujo, 2001). In one particular oil painting, he depicted himself not as a prisoner, but as an artist. There is no barbed wire or reference to the star Jews were forced to wear on their clothing; instead, the image is of Nussbaum at his easel painting on a canvas. Milton (2000) noted how this work, unlike his other self-portraits that emphasize his experience of oppression, affirms Nussbaum's identity as an artist.

A subcategory of portraiture is Nazi-commissioned works. This category of artwork differs in that it was created specifically for Nazi use and not out of the artists' own desire to create. Though the artists who produced these works did not have to do so in secret, the nature of the works was morally problematic. The artists were often tasked with creating propaganda posters disputing the realities of camps and ghettos (Green, 1978) or making art for Nazi enjoyment. In Auschwitz, Czech artist Dina Gottlibova was selected by notorious Nazi doctor Josef Mengele to paint portraits of the prisoners he used for genetic experimentations (Robinson, 2015). Dissatisfied with photographs, Mengele requested that Gottlibova pay extra attention to his victims' skin color, to show that they were an inferior race. Gottlibova demanded that her mother's life be spared as long as she was in the camp, to which Mengele agreed. Dreifuss-Kattan (2016) noted the contradiction Gottlibova experienced in being a witness to Mengele's evil, but also being spared a similar fate by being in his service. Through this commission, Gottlibova strived to commemorate the life of Mengele's victims while saving her own. In interviews, the artist has repeatedly stated that she relied on her ability to save her life (Costanza, 1983; Helstein, 2009).

A less documented story is that of Marianne Grant, who was also forced into drawing for Dr. Mengele's perverse experiments. Grant was assigned to draw portraits of twins and dwarfs, and recalled the jarring experience of working with Mengele by her side:

> He handed me an architect's tool set and I had to draw the family tree of one of the Hungarian dwarf families in black ink. He paced up and down in his high leather boots without a word. I was shaking. If I had made a blob or mistake I would have been finished. At this time I knew I was painting for my life (2002. p. 5).

Stationed in the artists' workshop at Terezín, Charolette Burseova was tasked with reproducing classic paintings for Nazi guards (Rosenberg, 2001). One guard was so impressed with her portrait of the Madonna that he advised her to never complete it; as long as the painting was in progress, Buresova would remain useful, rather than disposable like other ghetto residents. This commission ultimately kept her safe from deportation to the death camps. Burseova was one of the few residents of Terezín who was never sent on a transport to Auschwitz. She escaped the ghetto just three days before it was liberated in 1945 and returned to Prague.

These examples illustrate the Nazis' exploitation of their captives' talents. In each instance, the artist's skill rendered them useful and therefore worthy of living. At times, these artists even received additional rations of food as compensation for their efforts. These commissions kept them safe; but they were aware of the precarious nature of this work. Gottlibova and Grant both indicated that any mistake could have made them dispensable to Mengele. Still, Gottlibova, Grant, and Burseova all made unofficial art, in addition to their official commissioned works, at some point during their captivity. The portraits that remain, though commissioned for nefarious reasons, do pay homage to their subjects. Looking at the carefully rendered portraits commissioned by Nazis, viewers can appreciate the human life imbued in the artwork and mourn the loss of the subjects who were ultimately murdered. Gottlibova, Grant and Buresova can also be recognized for making their subjects, who were destined for death, so lifelike and individualized.

LANDSCAPES

Scenic views and depictions of artists' surroundings, such as landscapes and genre paintings, historically have been prominent subjects in European painting (Janson, Janson & Marmor, 1997), and continue to be relevant in contemporary studios. This preference persisted in the makeshift studios of camps and ghettos, as evidenced by depictions of nearby mountains, bodies of water and courtyards. The category of landscape artwork also includes architectural sketches of buildings and barracks drawn in front of nearby mountains or fields. Sujo (2001) suggested that images of mountains and sky represented both an escape from confinement and a survival instinct. Placing camp scenes, and subsequently the artist, against known images such as the Pyrenees mountains may have been an attempt to document where the camps were located. Including recognizable landmarks and even country flags further supported the desire to document and offer proof of where the artists were imprisoned.

Frankl (1959/2006) noted one such occasion for appreciating beauty when he described watching a sunset one evening in Auschwitz and remembered "how beautiful the world could be" (p. 40). It could be argued that the recognition of beauty served to assuage the artists' fears and restore a semblance of faith. This is a theme in the work of Karl Schwesig, who painted landscapes in multiple French internment camps. Many of his paintings appear to have been painted anywhere but an internment camp, and can even be described as peaceful, as they are characterized by bright skies and a soft brush stroke. Of Schwesig's work, Moreh-Rosenberg wrote: "despite the harsh conditions in captivity, he attempted through painting to capture a passing moment of enchantment" (2016, p. 246). Landscape drawings and paintings also allowed artists to address the contradiction between the splendor of nature and the grim realities of their living conditions. Shen-Dar (2003) noted that landscape paintings from the Gurs camp conveyed this polarity through the use of color. Artists such as Leo Breuer used dull grays, browns and black to depict internal areas of Gurs, such as the barracks and soil, while filling the sky and mountain range in the background with rich blues and purples (Figure 3.2).

This contradiction is evident in the writing of artist Yvonne Useldinger, who drew throughout her imprisonment in the female concentration camp Ravensbrück. In a journal entry she wrote:

> Today I saw something really special. A swan on the little pond offered a wonderful scene to draw. Nature here is always full of surprises. Although one always sees new wonders in the same view, the electrified barbed wire brings us quickly back to reality (as cited in Morrison, 2010, p. 159).

The drawing Useldinger described was likely destroyed; however, her words describe the paradox between natural beauty and the ugliness of the camp.

The reminder that the outside world continued to exist may have been another motivation for artists depicting landscapes. Terezín survivor Helga Pollack recalled art lessons with Friedl Dicker-Brandeis: "We would draw from the window the sky, the mountains, nature… That is probably especially important for prisoners: to see the world on the other side, to know that it exists" (as cited in Makarova, 2001, p. 214). Blatter and Milton (1981) described landscape images as "flights into a world of fantasy and memory" (p. 29). Perhaps drawing the outside world, a fantastical world that the artists had once been a part of, gave them a sense of hope that they would one day return to it. Knowing that the outside world continued to exist proved that not all of their past life had been obliterated.

In this vein, Milton (2000) believed that landscape artwork strengthened the artists' connection to their life outside of captivity. While interned in Auschwitz, Polish artist Bronislaw Czech exclusively drew images depicting the Tatra mountains where he was raised. Fellow inmate Jozef Cyrankiewicz recalled that Czech "was always pinning for his skis, the snow, for movement in the air of the high mountains" (as cited in Kosiec, 1989, p. 8). The importance of landscape imagery to a pre-war connection is also evident in the artwork of Francis Reisz, a Viennese artist who lived in Paris before his deportation to Auschwitz. His vibrant painting *Pont Marie in Paris* (Figure 3.3) shows a street corner next to the bridge over the Seine river. The colorful buildings and blooming trees suggest a brightness completely incongruent with the dark environment he was trapped in. Even more interesting is the contrast of this painting to the official drawings he was tasked with completing: the technical drawings of the crematoria (Kosiec, 1989). I was able to speak with Reisz's daughter briefly about his artwork. Although she was not familiar with his Auschwitz era paintings, she shared that he was known in his post-war life for his optimism. This quality, she assumed, motivated his personal work during captivity. By drawing scenes of beauty that he had previously been immersed in, he was able to transcend the dark circumstances that represented his current reality.

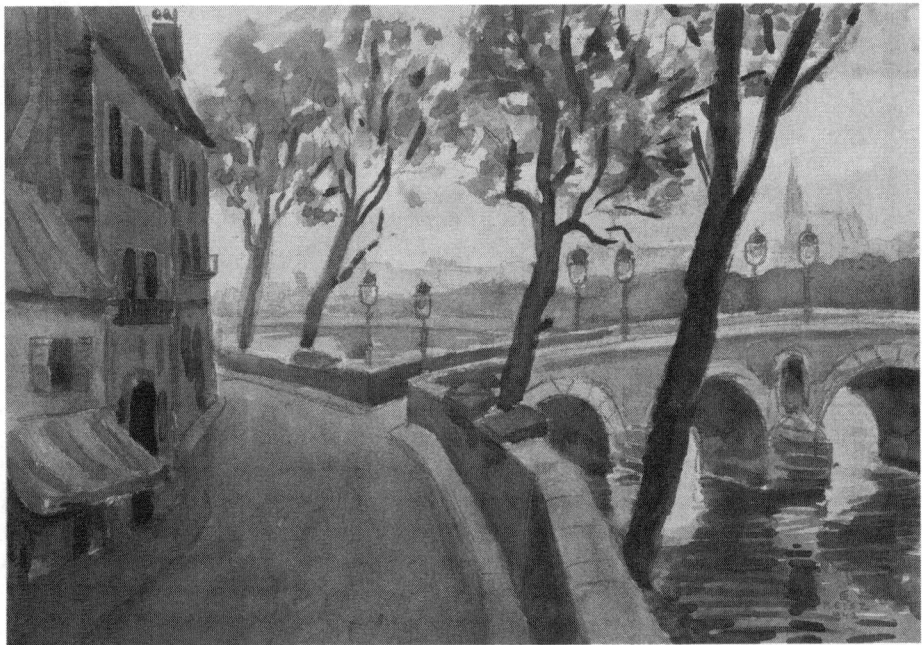

Figure 3.3 Francis Reisz (1909–1984). *Pont Marie in Paris*. Auschwitz 1942. Courtesy of the Auschwitz-Birkenau State Museum.

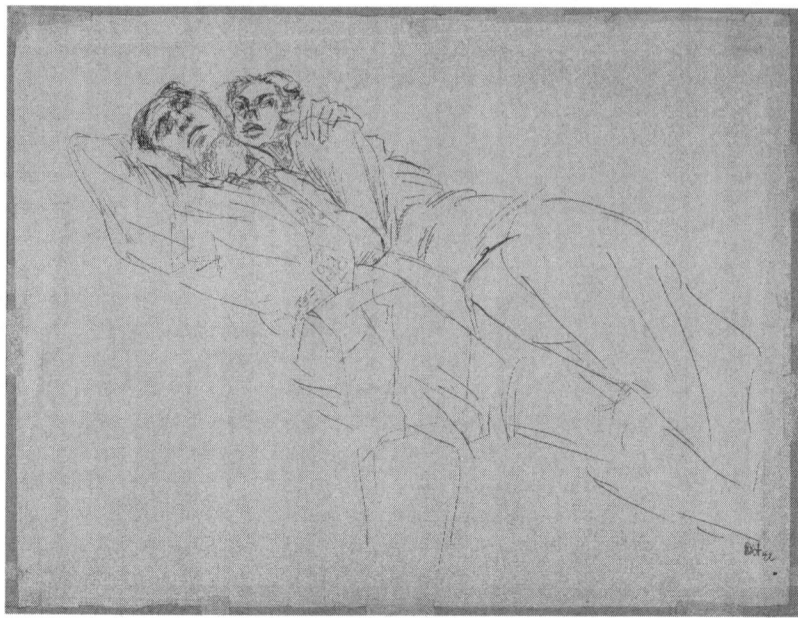

Figure 3.4 Lili Andrieux (1914–1996). *Together—For How Long?* Gurs camp, France, 1942. United States Holocaust Memorial Museum, courtesy of Lili Andrieux.

POSITIVE INTERACTIONS BETWEEN INMATES

The inhuman conditions in the ghettos and concentration camps at times resulted in conflict between prisoners. Levi (1986) described the ritualistic and protective ways in which prisoners split food rations, always concerned that one could be taken advantage of. Nomberg-Przytyk (1985) recalled a barbaric incident on a crowded transport to Ravensbrück in which female *kapos*[1] killed and removed other prisoners in order to grant themselves additional standing room. That lives were lost for the sake of an extra foot of space highlights the normalization of inhumanity in the fight for survival. Although the constant struggle for life resulted in cruelty, numerous drawings have been found which depict camaraderie and tenderness between prisoners, instead of adversity (Figure 3.4). Camaraderie allowed individuals to retain a sense of decency and benevolence (Davidov & Eisikovits, 2015); depictions of such bonds testify that these qualities remained intact. Kimor (2002) noted that works such as these convey a sense of closeness and genuine concern shared between inmates, as they depict the social normalcy of rapport and support.

Presidao's (2016) study of female Holocaust artwork underscores the comradery between female prisoners evidenced in artworks. Her designation of the *mutual assistance* (Baumel 1993; Presidao, 2016) that appears in female Holocaust artwork can be classified under themes of positive interactions. *Mutual assistance* refers to the sense of solidarity that female inmates built in order to garner support for one another.

---

1 *Kapos* is the term used for camp prisoners whom Nazis trusted and therefore assigned to supervise other prisoners. *Kapos* were forced into complicity under threat of death.

Presiado noted that women in camps developed surrogate families (2016) to aid one another as their own biological families dwindled. Artworks depicting female mutual assistance highlight areas seen as particular value to women (Bos, 2003; Ringelheim, 1985) including friendship, emotional support, bonding and trust. Presiado asserted that such themes demonstrate how female captives retained a sense of humanity and courage in a manner which fulfilled gender and cultural expectations (2016).

The comradery between women is evident in images created by a range of female artists. Many of these artworks exemplifying mutual assistance were produced in the Ravensbrück camp, as this was the only all-female concentration camp in operation. Jeannette L'Herminer, who was arrested for her participation in the French Resistance, made over 150 drawings and paintings while interned in Ravensbrück. The majority of her works depict a sense of bonding and support between captives. Her female figures are often rendered leaning against or physically supporting each other, illuminating the extent to which the prisoners of Ravensbrück relied on their peers (Presdiado, 2016). Of note, Ravensbrück was the site of medical experiments and a number of prisoners suffered dangerous operations on their legs, thus leaving them in need of physical support from fellow inmates. Helen Ernst's *Women of Ravensbrück*, which she created immediately after liberation, also illustrates the concept of mutual assistance. The painting features a group of women standing together in a tight room, holding hands. Their faces indicate they are in pain, but the mutual assistance between them is clear in their grasp on each other. On the left, one figure supports another who is visibly pregnant with a hug. According to Presidao, "these women transmit a sense of solidarity, despite the violent attempts to break their spirits" (2016, p. 9). Ernst's painting encapsulates the Ravensbrück prisoner experience. Through danger and cruelty, emotional support prevailed.

Many interactions included in this category of art depict participation in religious activities. Holocaust scholar David G. Roskies noted the strength of the Jewish traditions in ghetto cultural activity, as evidenced by the similarities across the Lodz, Warsaw, and Vilnius ghettos (2004). Much of the artwork that exists from Nazi ghettos illustrates this engagement. The majority of works showing religious activity were made in Terezín, as the observance of Jewish holidays and traditions was tolerated in the model ghetto. Karel Fleischmann drew four elders reading the *Torah* in Terezín. Green (1978) noted the inspiration and courage in Kleischmann's figures. Helga Hošková-Weissová drew the manager of the children's home in Terezín lighting *Hannukah* candles surrounded by children watching attentively. Her published diary reads: "The cramped loft space of L410 filled up with the figures of girls. The forst candle on the memorah flared into life and objects stretched into long, scary shadows. Three hundred and sixty pairs of eyes lit up" (Weiss, 2013, p. 117). These, and other drawings of Jewish cultural traditions, highlight the need to retain cultural values. By continuing to observe religious traditions and documenting them in drawings, ghetto residents maintained a hold on the very cultural identity that led them to captivity.

MEMORIES OF LIFE BEFORE

Lively, sometimes colorful images of life prior to the war affirmed a sense of hope and a determination to return to that reality. Langer deemed these works as documents of what was lost, rather than what was preserved (1995). In creating images of pre-captivity scenes and memories, artists paused to appreciate the small comforts of their past life. While hiding in Poland, six-year-old Nelly Toll painted watercolor scenes of a joyful, imaginative world (Moreh-Rosenberg, 2016). With her mother's encouragement, Toll combined memories of her past life with fairytale elements—a contrast to the war-torn city they had fled. Notably, Toll later emigrated to the United States and eventually completed a master's degree in art therapy at Hahnemann University in Philadelphia, now Drexel University. I was able to speak with her via phone in 2017 regarding my research, though she was unable to participate in my study (detailed in Part 2 of this text).

Terezín artist Bedrich Fritta created a picture book for his son's third birthday (Amishai-Maisels, 1993; Green, 1978), which depicted his hopes for a future life. Fritta began the book, *To Tommy, for His Third Birthday in Terezin, 22 January 1944*, with a cartoon Tommy peering out the ghetto window, then used watercolors to depict lively scenes of a bright and fulfilling life. The book contains imagined drawings of Tommy eating ice cream, ice skating and traveling the world—all memories that Fritta had, which he hoped would be a part of his son's future. Tommy wasn't even one year old when his family entered the ghetto, so the artwork became a representation of what Fritta wanted for, but couldn't provide, his son. The book was hidden in the ghetto and given to Tommy after the war by his adopted father, Leo Haas, who had worked in the technical department with Fritta. An adult Tommy reflected on the significance of the book at a 2013 exhibit of his father's Terezín artwork in Berlin: "The only thing that remains to me, that belongs to me, that was made for me alone, is my book, a book by my father. In that book I can feel him, his tears, his hope, his fear" (2013). Although the book was intended for a child, the images are Fritta's attempts to preserve the memories of his life outside of the ghetto.

In a testimonial, Auschwitz artist Mieczyslaw Koscieelniak explained his need to draw non-camp scenes: "The further subjects were born from memories and yearning. They were imagined works... It was self-defense-the flight of the psyche from the horrifying reality in which I had to live being an Auschwitz inmate" (as cited in Sieradzka, 2019). The collection of Koscieeelniak's drawings owned by the Aushwitz-Birkenau State Museum includes mostly raw, dark scenes emphasizing the brutality of camp life. However, his words indicate that he occasionally made the choice to psychically escape his surroundings and draw representations of his life before imprisonment (Sieradzka, 2019.).

DEPICTIONS OF BRUTALITY

The aforementioned categories of artwork suggest that some artists were able to transcend their bleak surroundings by creating artworks representing beauty, human connection and fond memories. Other artists felt a strong need to document the obscene conditions that comprised their reality by drawing the violence, death and destruction around them in order to "depict the genocidal impulse that was beyond the imagination" (Langer, 1996, p. 59). Milton (2000) referred to these images as "evidentiary art" (p. 91), as they serve as evidence of the hunger, despair, sickness and cruelty that were omnipresent in ghetto and camp life. Artworks in this category range from documentations of mass despair to individual frailty. Some works show the routine scenes of daily roll calls, selections and forced labor that have become generic depictions of camp and ghetto life; while others images depict a single corpse, forcing the viewer to consider the individual suffering within the mass suffering (Milton, 2000).

Drawing these and other disturbing scenes of daily life may have represented an attempt to reconcile or make sense of the surreal environment. Of note, while these abysmal scenes represented a constant reality, this particular category of art is the smallest in the Auschwitz museum collection. Curators at the Auschwitz museum believe this is because if they had been discovered, such scenes would have put the artist at greater risk than lighter, more innocuous drawings. The Nazis were careful not to expose the reality of life in the camps. Even Auschwitz commandant Rudolph Hoss forbade Germans from taking photographs inside the camp.

To record the terrors of camps and ghettos for the outside world, Auschwitz survivor Mieczysław Kościelniak (Figure 3.5) drew scenes of weak prisoners returning from work duties, men standing in line for roll calls, beatings and hunger. Kościelniak's drawings encompass a large amount of the Auschwitz art collection. In a testimony, the artist stated: "My eagerness to record the events in the camp commenced some time in 1942. It was then that I sketched the bodies of colleagues lying by the camp kitchen" (as cited in Sieradzka, 2019).

Some artists, such as a group employed in the Terezín technical department, were motivated to use art to document their experiences (Green, 1978) in the hope that their works would be discovered and serve as evidence against Nazi perpetrators. Because of this, most works in this category are rendered realistically. Boris Taslitzki's drawings feature frail, naked Buchenwald prisoners on the brink of death.

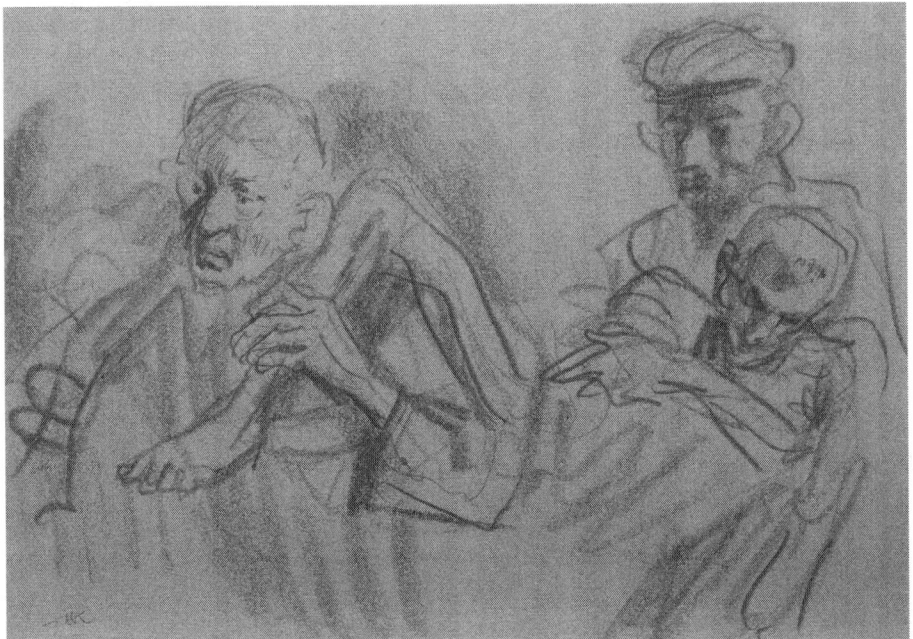

Figure 3.5 Mieczysław Kościelniak (1912–1993). *Friendly Favour.* Auschwitz, 1943. Brown crayon, paper, 21 × 29.5 cm. Printed with permission from the Auschwitz-Birkenau State Museum.

Leon Delarbre's series from Dora show hanged men detailed with their hands tied behind their backs and wood blocks in their mouths to muffle their cries (Delarbre, 1945). In his role as a block monitor at the Birkenau hospital, Polish artist Waldemar Nowakowski witnessed multiple starvation deaths, which he documented in his drawings (Dalek & Swiebocka, 1989).

Other artists used a more symbolic approach to convey the death and disparity. Simon Wiesenthal, who after liberation relentlessly pursued Nazis in hiding, drew trains pulling into Mathhauseen, where he was imprisoned. Instead of drawing barracks or a crematorium, as other artists did in pictures of the transports, Wiesenthal depicted the trains entering the mouth of a skull wearing a Nazi uniform hat, symbolizing how the majority of passengers on the train were brought to their deaths. In his drawing *Roll Call*, Jozef Szajna depicted the seemingly endless experience of standing for roll call at Buchenwald with simplified figures articulated by striped uniforms and bald heads. Each figure seems to blend into the next, highlighting how unrecognizable the prisoners had become. A number of pieces feature a Nazi guard exaggerated to a large size, with prisoners drawn as tiny and insignificant in comparison, showing the lack of power prisoners had. These symbolic works serve to document the artists' experience, while also conveying the mood of the setting.

SATIRICAL WORKS

In contrast to the harrowing, realistic works, some artists experimented with humor and satire. Surviving artist Wiktor Siminski considered himself the camp cartoonist as he drew stylized postcards of daily scenes from Sachsenhausen (Cognet, 2013). According to survivor Viktor Frankl, "the attempt to develop a sense of humor and to see things in a humorous light is some kind of a trick learned while mastering the art of living" (1959/2006, p.44). Even with the abundance of violence and brutality, some artists responded to the abysmal conditions in camp systems and ghettos with humor. Morreall (2009) noted that although the topic of the Holocaust is far from humorous, humor served three functions for Holocaust victims:

> First was a critical function: humor focused attention on what was wrong and sparked resistance to it. Second was its cohesive function; it created solidarity in those laughing together at the oppressors. And third was its coping function: it helped the oppressed get through their suffering without going insane. (p. 119)

An example of artwork providing a critical function of humor can be found in *Mickey Mouse in the Gurs Internment Camp* by artist Horst Rosenthal. In this 12-page comic style booklet, Rosenthal draws the cartoon figure in daily scenes from the camp, supplementing the illustrations with text spoken by Mickey, which expressed Rosenthal's point of view. In her discussion of the artist's work, Rosenberg (2002) emphasized the contradiction between Mickey Mouse (a symbol of innocence and freedom) and the harsh realities of camp life. Rosenthal, who had left his native Poland to seek refuge in France, used Mickey Mouse to represent himself in this autobiographical account of his experience. The story begins with Mickey smiling, enjoying his freedom in France. Suddenly, Mickey is arrested: "A gendarme approached me... 'Son of a b**, your papers!' Papers? I never had any. I am paperless. I am international! 'Ah! A foreigner! Right, come with me to the station.' And so I found myself in Gurs!!'" (Rosenberg, 2002, p. 277).

Rosenthal's story continues as Mickey experiences the tension of bread distribution among prisoners and the censorship of mail by guards. Mickey remains positive as he demonstrates resourcefulness, a reflection of Rosenthal's own resilience during his internment. Since Rosenthal could not predict how his own story would end, he allowed Mickey to live out his fantasy of escaping with the decision to "erase myself" (in Rosenberg, 2002, p. 278).

Rosenthal's second and third booklets—*A Small Guide Through Gurs Camp 1942* and A *Day in the Life of a Resident, Gurs Internment Camp, 1942,* respectively—are satirical in nature. Idealistic scenes of prisoners and guards are drawn in a cartoon-like manner, with blunt text addressing the lack of food and unsanitary conditions. Rosenberg commented that these three stories do not include the violence or brutality that was common in Gurs. Instead, they highlight the injustice of being imprisoned. Each booklet references the "arbitrary bureaucracy" (Rosenberg, 2002, p. 286) that resulted in prisoners' illogical internment. Rosenthal seems to have been fueled by his disillusionment of the French government, and uses the three booklets to reconcile the unsettling and daunting place he found himself in.

Satirical and humorous artworks strengthened the cohesion of those in captivity, as it allowed them to share their experiences in a social, almost enjoyable way. An anonymous survivor testified:

> Even in the most difficult conditions and apparently hopeless situations, the impact of people with an outstanding sense of humor on the camp's community gave a realistic opportunity for even a temporary sustenance in the camp to the at risk and morally disturbed individuals (as cited in Jagoda, Kłodziński & Masłowski, 1981, p. 155).

Survivor Jerzy Rawicz stated: "Humor was an important weapon for the inmates. It saved us from breaking down" (as cited in Jagoda, Kłodziński & Masłowski, 1981, p. 150). Humor as a coping mechanism is evident in artworks from Auschwitz and other camps and ghettos. Inmates in Auschwitz drew caricatures of their captors, including *Kapos* and SS guards, which they shared secretly with each other (Sieradzka, 2019). These unflattering caricatures served to undermine the authority of the captures and even drew laughter out of prisoners. As Gussak states: "using humor in a horrific situation, the powerless gain strength and the powerful are made impotent" (2022).

Artist Friedl Dicker Brandeis, who drew with children in the Terezín ghetto, was known to address her situation with humor, at least prior to her transport to Terezín. An old friend recalled visiting Friedl in the Czech countryside soon after the German occupation: "she grabbed a spool of black thread, stuck it under her nose and gave a congratulatory speech as Hitler. We were all doubled over with laughter" (as cited in Makarova, 2001, p. 25).

In addition to the aforementioned functions of humor in Holocaust art, Feinstein (2008) added the function of resistance, as satirical works demonstrated a resistance against the Nazi regime. Most of the artwork I have described can be classified as a form of resistance, though satirical artworks illuminate the concept of resistance, as they demonstrate victims' ability to maintain a sense of humor and not be completely broken down by oppression.

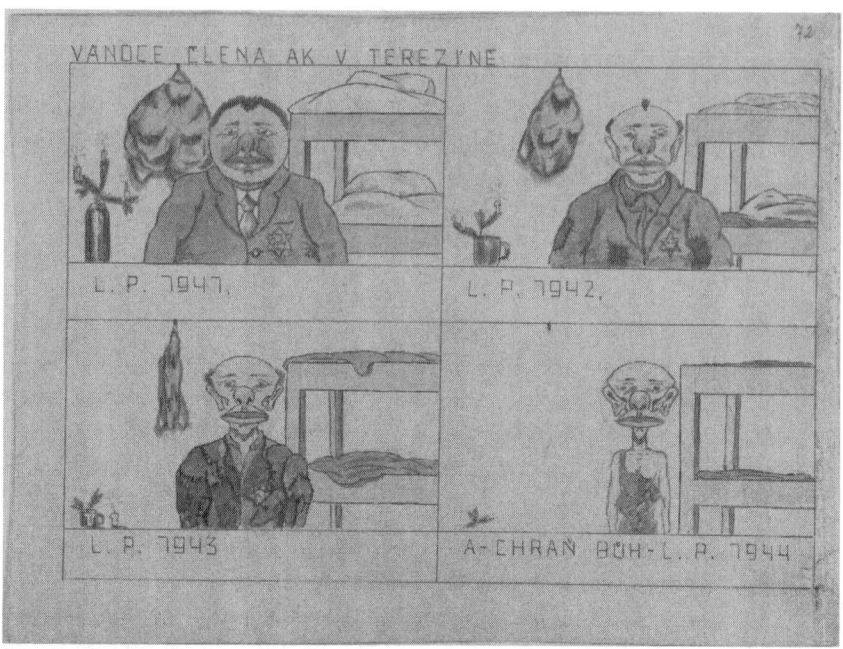

Figure 3.6 Pavel Fantl (1903–1945). *Metamorphosis.* Theresienstadt ghetto, 1944. Watercolor, pencil and India ink on paper, 22.8 × 29.7 cm. Collection of the Yad Vashem Art Museum, Jerusalem. Gift of Ida Fantlová, the artist's mother, courtesy of Ze'ev and Alice Shek, Caesarea, Israel. Photo © Yad Vashem Art Museum, Jerusalem.

Caricatures, which were often drawn to celebrate birthdays and holidays, were also common in camp art. Explained Dalek & Swiebocka (1989):

> If we accept that caricature expresses a keen evaluation of reality, that it thrives on contradictions and finally, that exaggeration is the method of the cartoonist, distorting human traits thing, and events, in fact showing the world in a distorting mirror, then no wonder it was popular among the concentration camp artists. Auschwitz was a world totally distorted, black and white, without half tones, in which the boundary between light and darkness, good and evil were clearly drawn, where to declare oneself on the side of elementary human values often meant passing to the domain of death (p. 7).

Czech physician Pavel Fantl was known for making dozens of satirical drawings and caricatures during his time in the Terezín ghetto. His drawing *Metamorphosis* (Figure 3.6) presents as a comic strip. In four squares, Fantl illustrated the effects of starvation and manual labor on a Terezín inmate. The individual appears to be deteriorating, losing weight, hair and color. His belongings in the background are also reduced, further indicating how conditions worsened over time in the ghetto.

CONCLUSIONS

The categories I have laid out in this chapter help me to make the art of the Holocaust more approachable. By examining it beyond the graphic and shocking imagery we can grasp the nuances that the artists took into consideration. Distinguishing categories of artwork illuminates the motivation for each piece. This allows us to conceptualize the artists not solely as helpless victims, but as individuals driven by a greater desire. In each of these categories of artwork, there is evidence of the transformational power of creativity. Artists created works authentically as a means of savoring dignity, restoring hope and affirming identity. Though in many instances the risks were great, the need to create was somehow greater. Making art allowed camp and ghetto inhabitants to retain a tenuous grasp on their humanity and transcend their environments to find a sense of meaning. They responded to their situation through art. Alexander Bogen (as cited in Costanza, 1982) stated: "Each man, when standing face to face with cruel danger, with death, reacts in his own way. The artist reacts with his means. This is his protest! This is my means! He reacts in an artistic way" (p. xvii).

Categorizing the art created during the Holocaust illuminates the individuality and humanity of those who suffered. The artwork serves as a reminder that those targeted by Nazi oppression were humans, capable of creation and expression. It forces viewers to recognize the individuals who suffered within a mass genocide (Leclerc, 2011), and appeals to us on relational and interpersonal levels. Through these categories of art, we recognize a capacity for resilience as well as a discovery of meaning. The artists discussed in this chapter found ways to make their grim realities worth surviving.

REFERENCES

Amishai-Maisels, Z. (1993). *Depiction and interpretation: The influence of the Holocaust on visual arts.* Tarrytown, NY: Pergamon Press.

Baumel, J. T. (1993). The 'Zehnerschaft' as an example of mutual assistance among women during the Holocaust. *Dapim: Studies on the Holocaust, 10,* 107–128.

Benvenuti, A. (2017). *Imprisoned: Drawings from Nazi concentration camps.* New York, NY: Skyhorse.

Blatner, J. & Milton, S. (1981). *Art of the Holocaust.* New York, NY: Routledge.

Bohm-Duchen, M. (2013). Creativity against all odds: Art and internment during World War II. In P. Tame, D. Jeannerod, & M. Braganca (Eds.), *Mnemosyne and Mars: Artistic and cultural representations of twentieth-century Europe at war* (pp. 183–201). London, England: Cambridge Scholars.

Bos, P.R. Women and the Holocaust: Analyzing gender difference. In E.R Baer and M. Goldberg (Eds.). *Experience and expression: Women, the Nazis and the Holocaust,* 23–50. Detroit, MI: Wayne State University Press, 2003.

Cognet, C. (Director/writer/producer). (2014). *Because I was a painter* (Motion Picture). United States: Cinema Guild.

Costanza, M. (1982). *The living witness: Art in the concentration camps and ghettos.* New York, NY: The Free Press.

Davidov, J. & Eisikovits, Z. (2015). Free will in total institutions: The case of choice inside Nazi death camps. *Consciousness and Cognition, 34,* 87–97. doi:10.1016/j.concog.2015.03.018

Dalek, J. & Swiebocka, T. (1989) *Suffering and hope: Artistic creations of the Oświęcim Prisoners* (J. Kosiec, trans.). Oświęcim, Poland: Panstwowe Muzeum Auschwitz-Birkenau.

Delarbre, L. (1945). *Dora, Auschwitz, Buchenwald, Bergen-Belsen: Croquis clandestins.* Paris, France: M. de Romilly.

Dreifuss-Kattan, E. (2016). *Art and mourning: The role of creativity in healing trauma and loss.* New York, NY: Routledge.

Felstiner, M.L. Charlotte Salomon. *Shalvi/Hyman encyclopedia of Jewish women*. 31 December 1999. Jewish Women's Archive. https://jwa.org/encyclopedia/article/salomon-charlotte.

Frankl, V. (1959/2006). *Man's search for meaning* (5th ed.) (I. Lasch, Trans.). Boston, MA: Beacon Press.

Grant, M. (2002). *I knew I was painting for my life: The Holocaust artworks of Marianne Grant*. Glasgow, Scotland: Glasgow Museums.

Green, G. (1978). *The artists of Terezin*. New York, NY: Hawthorn Books.

Gussak, D. (2022). *The frenzied dance of art and violence*. New York, NY: Oxford University Press.

Helstein, H. (Director/writer/producer). (2008). *As seen through these eyes* (Motion Picture). United States: Parkchester Pictures.

Jagoda Z., Kłodziński S., Masłowski J. (1981). *Oświęcim Nieznany*. Krakow, Poland: Wydawnictwo Literackie.

Janson, H. W., Janson, A. F., & Marmor, M. (1997). *History of art*. London, England: Thames and Hudson.

Kalmanowitz, D., & Lloyd, B. (2004). *Art therapy and political violence: With art, without illusion*. New York, NY: Routledge.

Kantor, A. (1971). *The book of Alfred Kantor: An artist's journal of the Holocaust*. New York, NY: McGraw Hill.

Kimor, E. (2002). The women's voice. *Jewish Quarterly*, *49*(3), 27–29. doi: 10.1080/0449010X.2002.10706788

Langer, L. (1996). *Admitting the Holocaust: Collected essays*. New York, NY: Oxford University Press.

Leclerc, J. (2011). Re-presenting trauma: The witness function in the art of the Holocaust. *Art Therapy*, *28*(2), 82–89, doi: 10.1080/07421656.2011.580181

Levi, P. (1986) *The drowned and the saved*. New York, NY: Summit Books

Makarova, E. (2001). *Friedl Dicker-Brandeis*. Los Angeles, CA: Tallfellow/Ever Picture Press.

Milton, S. (2000). Culture under duress: Art and the Holocaust. In F. C. Decoste and B. Schwartz (Eds.). *The Holocaust's ghost: Writings on art, politics, law and education*. Edmonton, AB: University of Alberta Press, 84–96.

Moreh-Rosenberg, E. (2012). *Last portrait*. http://www.yadvashem.org/yv/en/exhibitions/last_portrait/overview.asp.

Moreh-Rosenberg, E. (2016). *The art from the Holocaust*. Cologne, Germany: Wienand Verlag.

Morreall, J. (2009). *Comic relief: A comprehensive philosophy of humor*. Hoboken, NJ: Wiley Blackwell.

Morrison, J. G. (2000). *Ravensbrück: Everyday life in a women's concentration camp. 1939-45*. Princeton, NJ: Markus Wiener Publishers.

Nomberg-Przytyk, S. (1985). *Auschwitz: True tales from a grotesque land*. Chapel Hill, NC: The University of North Carolina Press.

Presiado, M. (2016). A new perspective on Holocaust art: women's artistic expression of the female Holocaust experience (1939–49), *Holocaust Studies*, *22*(4), 417–446. doi:10.1080/17504902.2016.1201365

Ringelheim, J. (1985). Women and the Holocaust: A reconsideration of research. *Signs: Journal of Women in Culture and Society*, *10*(4), 741–761.

Robinson, N. (2015). Snow White in Auschwitz: The tale of Dina Gottliebova-Babbit. In *Working memory: women and work in World War II*. (pp. 129–152). Waterloo, ON: Wilfrid Laurier University Press.

Rosenberg, P. (2009, March). Art during the Holocaust. *Jewish Women's Archive*. http://jwa.org/encyclopedia/article/art-during-holocaust

Roskies, D. G. (2004). Jewish cultural life in the Vilna ghetto and in Lithuania and the Jews. *The Holocaust chapter: Symposium presentations*. Washington, D.C.: The United States Holocaust Memorial Museum, 33–44.

Shen-Dar, Y. (2003). Victory for the creative spirit behind barbed wire. In B. Gutterman & N. Morgenstern (Eds.). *The Gurs Haggadah: Passover in perdition* (N. Kanner, Trans., pp. 95–101). Jerusalem, Israel: Devora.

Sieradzka, A. (2019). *Art at Auschwitz*. http://lekcja.auschwitz.org/en_18_sztuka/ Oświęcim: Państwowe Muzeum Auschwitz-Birkenau/Auschwitz-Birkenau State Museum

Steinberg, M. P. & Bohm-Duchen, M. (2006). *Reading Charlotte Salomon*. Ithaca, NY: Cornell University Press.

Stiftung Neue Synagogue Berlin – Centrum Judaicum and Museumspädagogiischen Dienst Berlin. (2005). *Art in Auschwitz 1940–1945 exhibit* [Brochure]. Berlin, Germany: Rasch Verlag, Bramsche.

Sujo, G. (2001). *Legacies of silence: The visual arts and Holocaust memory*. London, England: Philip Wilson Publishers.

Szymańska, I. (1989). *Suffering and hope. Artistic works of prisoners of the Auschwitz camp*. Oświęcim, Poland: Publication Department of the Auschwitz Birkenau State Museum.

Weis, H. (2013). *Helga's diary: A young girl's account of life in a concentration camp*. New York, NY: W.W. Norton.

CHAPTER 4

ARTS CONTRIBUTING TO COMMUNITY

Although many artists worked independently, particularly in concentration camp systems, a number of artists created communally, developing a culture of creative engagement. The collective art of the Holocaust can serve as a reminder of how the arts can support and sustain the health of a community.

The brutality of the Holocaust necessitated healing at both personal and collective levels. Victims suffered not only as individuals, but also as members of a community. The Nazis targeted all European Jews as a singular group. They also directed their aggressions against homosexuals[1], Romani gypsies, Jehovah's Witnesses, and other non-dominant groups. Because these communities were besieged and almost completely annihilated, their suffering was also communal.

The idea that art making can bolster a community facing adversity is discussed in the art therapy literature. Ottemiller and Awais (2016) described the art process as one that can heal communities in need and generate change. According to Kapitan, Litell and Torres (2011), "a traumatized community may turn to the arts to help its members move from personal tragedy toward shared experiences that restore collective identity" (p. 65). Similar responses were evidenced by artists in select camps and ghettos who developed a sense of family and cohesion through making art collectively. Frederick Terna, who began his artistic career in Terezín, explained the impetus for a creative community: "They were maintaining a culture, a civilization, that had collapsed around them. Outside there was murder and mayhem, but inside it was different" (F. Terna, personal communication, September 5, 2017).

The notion of artwork emerging from camps and ghettos is inherently paradoxical: art making is a form of creative construction, which contradicts the goal of destruction typically associated with such environments. Indeed, "a waiting room for the horrors of the death camps seems an unlikely setting for something meant to liberate the spirit and bring it joy" (Bak, 2001, p. 20). And yet artwork was not only produced in these vile conditions, but occasionally exhibited and celebrated.

In this chapter, I detail select examples of art making as it bolstered community and led to a degree of communal healing within camps and ghettos. I cite examples from Nazi ghettos, internment camps, and concentration camps, including Terezín, Vilna, Gurs, St. Cyprien, Ravensbrück and Auschwitz. I then discuss the topic of community art making from an art therapy perspective to further highlight the parallels between contemporary art therapy practices and the Holocaust art phenomenon. I propose that the communal art making that occurred in Nazi camps and ghettos can exemplify the benefits described in art therapy literature. It also lends credence to community art practices as an opportunity to heal and empower marginalized communities.

TEREZÍN

In 1941, the small town of Terezín was evacuated to serve as a Nazi ghetto. Terezín—or Theresienstadt, as the Germans called it—is located 60 kilometers northwest of Prague. An estimated 150,000 total prisoners passed through Terezín during WWII,

DOI: 10.4324/9781003160885-6

mostly on their way to Auschwitz. Though primarily a ghetto, Terezín's interior Small Fortress served as an actual prison, where law-breaking residents of the ghetto were sent to be tortured or killed.

Nazi propaganda depicted Terezín in a way that covered up the Nazi plan for its "Final Solution." Joseph Goebbels, minister of Nazi propaganda (as cited in Makarova, 2001), said: "While the Jews in Theresienstadt sit in cafes drinking coffee, eating cake and dancing, our soldiers bear all the weight of a horrible war" (p. 29). Terezín served as the backdrop for various propaganda films produced by the Third Reich Ministry of Propaganda, including *The Fuhrer Gives a Town to the Jews.* In 1943, the Nazis erected shops in Terezín's main square, which sold goods taken from the prisoners. The shops—along with a post office, bank and coffee house—were all part of an illusory town square. When Red Cross representatives came to investigate Terezín, the Nazis made sure that only the healthiest residents of the town were seen in public.

Because Terezín was used as a model ghetto, the restrictions on cultural activities were inconsistent. Nazi guards allowed some cultural activities, which contributed to the overall guise of Terezín as a Jewish settlement (Dutlinger, 2001). At times, ghetto residents were permitted to engage in visual and performing arts; at other times, those acts were strictly prohibited. Survivor Alfred Kantor (1971) wrote about the paradox of life in Terezín: "One night, a brilliant cabaret in the cellar; the next, a transport leaving the station. I began to feel the need to record these bizarre scenes" (1971, para. 16). The transports Kantor referenced were cattle cars filled beyond capacity with Terezín residents, directed toward Auschwitz. Survivors I have spoken with noted that cultural activities were occasionally permitted directly prior to large transports to death camps. The guards provided a false sense of ease and comfort, as they allowed ghetto residents to engage in such humanizing activities before sending them to their deaths.

With this paradoxical environment, Terezín is known for having a vast artistic culture (Dutlinger, 2001; Langer, 1996). Theatrical performances, concerts and regular drawing lessons brought ghetto inhabitants together in a form of cultural resistance. Langer (1996) credited this activity with providing a sense of inviolability and sanctity in an uncertain environment. Composer Victor Ullmann, who participated in the ghetto's cultural activities, explained the motivation for creativity: "By the rivers of Babylon, there we sat – but by no means wept... our endeavors in the arts were commensurate with our will to live" (as cited in Spenser, 2001. p. 55).

Some of Europe's most talented artists, performers and musicians were prisoners at Terezín (Dutlinger, 2001). Recognizing this talent at their disposal, Terezín guards employed artists (organized into design departments) to create Nazi propaganda. These appointments offered certain amenities, such as extra rations of food and exemption from exhaustive labor, although the commissioned artists were prisoners and were treated as such. As a means of challenging that helplessness and fear, artists in Terezín used their talent as a silent form of resistance. When not under close watch, they created works depicting actual life in the ghetto (Figure 4.1). Knowing that this kind of work was prohibited and that producing it could lead to extreme punishment or death, they carefully hid their art. Green (1978) explained that by doing so, artists "kept alive not only the glowing embers of creativity, but did not shy from making their art a weapon" (p. 77). In July 1944, the clandestine artwork drawn in the design department was discovered by the Nazis and the artists responsible were

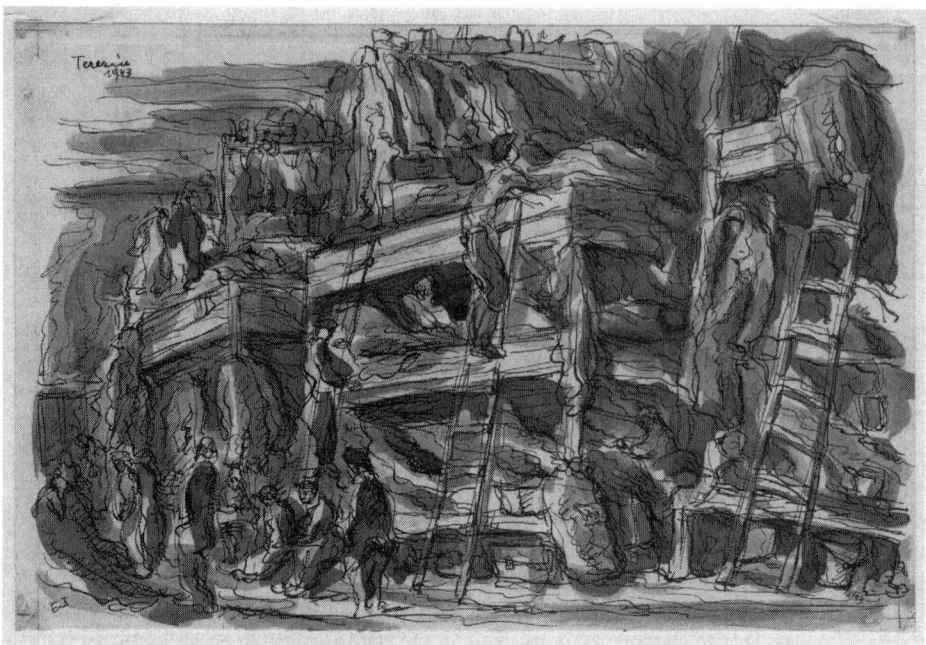

Figure 4.1 Karel Fleischmann (1897–1944). *Living Quarters—Sudeten Kaserne.* Theresienstadt ghetto, 1943. India ink and wash on paper, 22.5 × 33.2 cm. Collection of the Yad Vashem Art Museum, Jerusalem. Gift of the Prague Committee for Documentation, courtesy of Ze'ev and Alice Shek, Caesarea, Israel. Photo © Yad Vashem Art Museum, Jerusalem.

accused of projecting falsehoods. They were immediately sent to the Small Fortress with their families, where they were tortured for three months before being transported to death camps.

Another example of creative culture within the Terezín ghetto is the story of Bauhaus-educated artist Friedl Dicker-Brandeis, who set up art classes for children living in Terezín. When she learned that she would be sent to Terezín in 1942, she packed art materials to take with her. She anticipated finding children in the ghetto who would be in need of an outlet for expression. Upon arriving at Terezín, Dicker-Brandeis was assigned to work in the technical department with other artists. Displeased with this assignment, she requested a position at the girls' home, known as L 410, where she would eventually teach art and also live. Although art classes for children were not specifically prohibited, participation in them carried serious risks if discovered (Dutlinger, 2001). Still, Dicker-Brandeis worked within the existing parameters to engage the children in her care through art. In a letter, she explained the goals of her classes (as cited in Makarova, 2001):

> The drawing classes are not meant to make artists out of all the children. They are free to broaden such sources of energy as creativity and independence, to awaken the imagination, to strengthen the children's powers of observation and appreciation of reality. (p. 31)

The art classes gave the children a sense of cohesion and allowed for communal expression and interconnectedness in an otherwise isolating environment. After viewing an exhibit Dicker-Brandeis organized of the children's work, Terezín's director of child welfare, Egon Redlich (as cited in Makarova, 2001), commented: "The problems of Theresienstadt have found expression in the children's drawings" (p. 32).

Now a museum, Terezín holds a permanent exhibit of prisoner artwork. A sign in the museum reads: "In reality, cultural life became a powerful encouragement for the prisoners, giving them optimism and strength to resist demoralization. It was one of the most expressive manifestations of spiritual resistance."

VILNA GHETTO

While the culture of Terezín is well documented, artist communities also formed in other camp systems and ghettos. Vilna, Lithuania was a city known for creativity centuries before WWII, "where tradition and innovation harmoniously mingled" (Beinfeld, 2011, p. 94). Given this reputation, it is not surprising that artistic activity continued even after German troops seized control of Vilna. In June 1941, Germany occupied Vilna and instituted anti-Jewish decrees. Over the next few months, the German *Einsatzgruppe* routinely rounded up and executed mass groups of Vilna residents. By September 1941, the Germans had formally established a ghetto in Vilna. The imprisoned inhabitants of the ghetto were forced to live in overcrowded apartments. The adults among them had to work in factories or on manual labor sites outside the ghetto. Trunk noted that: "one is often tempted not to believe that such colorful, almost 'normal' cultural work took place in a ghetto where remnants of a decimated community were concentrated, constantly in danger of destruction" (1972, p. 219).

In 1943, artists in the Vilna ghetto organized an exhibition in order to maintain a sense of culture. Nine-year-old Samuel Bak was the only child invited to participate in the exhibition. At age 84, Bak discussed the importance of an art exhibit in the ghetto:

> People were somehow put in a situation in which they were victims of dehumanization. And within this fear in which they lived, they wanted to fight it, and humanize themselves as much as possible. Out of respect for the things that they thought were important in human life, that makes us more than animals. Appreciation of music, appreciation of literature, of visual arts, and so on, to give it importance. And it is not perchance that it happened within the sphere of the ghetto theater. Musicians were playing jazz, can you imagine, people playing jazz in the ghetto. But they were doing it because these were the moments when people were kind of allowed to become humans. (S. Bak, personal communication, October 10, 2017).

Bak's artwork in the Vilna ghetto was actually the start of his artistic career. He continued to draw and paint in a displaced persons camp following liberation, and eventually attended the Bezalel Academy of Arts and Design in Jerusalem. Bak has worked as a professional artist for most of his adult life. His post-war works deal with his memories of the Holocaust.

Another artist who was briefly involved in the Vilna ghetto's cultural community was Alexander Bogen. A native of Vilna and a trained artist, Bogen quickly acquainted himself with other artists in the ghetto. In an interview published on the website of

Yad Vashem, he recalled a strong desire to create—a desire that he and his fellow artists shared despite their precarious circumstances:

> I asked myself: 'Damn it, how is it that when I look – not at myself, but at the prospect of certain extermination – how can this be? How is it possible that in a person about to die this yearning for artistic expression is stronger than life?' (Yad Vashem, 2021).

Bogen described the cultural activity in the ghetto as "a dissonance to me" (Yad Vashem, n.d.). He believed that Jacob Gens, the head of the Vilna ghetto *Judenrat*, encouraged theater, art and music as an attempt to distract residents and give them a sense of comfort and calm. In 1943, Bogen escaped the ghetto and joined a group of Soviet partisans in the Narocz forests of Belarus. The partisans planned covert attacks on the Germans and eventually infiltrated the Vilna ghetto. Throughout his association with the partisans, Bogen kept sketching:

> All the time, in impossible conditions, I had a pencil and some paper, and I drew. When we would get back from a mission and sit by the campfire, drinking vodka and recounting the details of what happened, I would sit and draw the people, their experiences, and their clothes. I always had lots of drawings in my bag (Yad Vashem, n.d.).

Bogen may have been the only one of the partisans to draw during their downtime. However, his craft reinforced the comradery within the brigade. He recalled how Russian partisans requested him to draw their portraits. The Russians, he said, had a high regard for art. The portraits of his fellow partisans allowed him to connect with individuals from a different culture. Moreover, his personal values as an artist had resonated with others.

ST. CYPRIEN AND GURS

The St. Cyprien internment camp opened in February 1939 on the coast of France just north of the Spanish border. The first prisoners were Spanish refugees; though by the summer of 1940—after Germany invaded Belgium—refugees of French, German, Austrian and Belgian nationality were held captive in St. Cyprien. Artists imprisoned in the St. Cyprien internment camp were active during their captivity. The Red Cross and other relief organizations provided limited quantities of art supplies, such as watercolors, paper and pencils. French officials allowed art making since it kept the prisoners occupied. Artwork was traded among prisoners and guards for food, clothing and less rigorous work assignments (Milton, 2000). In addition to the supplies available, artists used driftwood and clay, and painted directly on the inside of canvas tents (Stein, 2013). In October 1940, a storm ravaged the camp and prisoners were transferred to other French internment camps; the majority were sent to Gurs (Rosenberg, 2001).

Located near the Pyrenees mountains, Gurs served as an internment and transit camp under the Vichy regime in France (United States Holocaust Memorial Museum, n.d.). Approximately 22,000 prisoners passed through Gurs between 1940 and 1943. The prisoners had to contend with shortages of food and water, and a looming uncertainty regarding their futures. In an attempt to retain their dignity and humanity, the artists imprisoned at Gurs focused on their creative endeavors whenever possible (Figure 4.2). Beginning in the fall of 1940, prisoners transformed one barracks in each block of Gurs into a "cultural center" for performances, lectures and

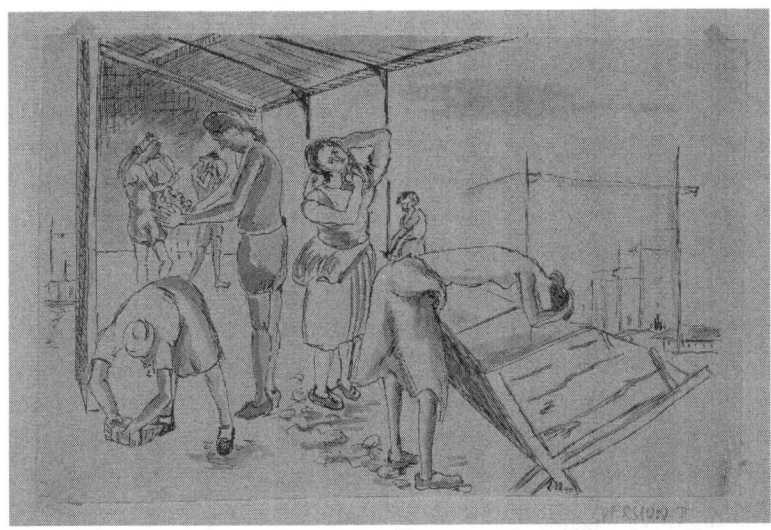

Figure 4.2 Lili Andrieux (1914–1996). *Women Washing Themselves II.* Gurs camp, France, 1940. United States Holocaust Memorial Museum, courtesy of Lili Andrieux.

art exhibits (Rosenberg, 2002; Shen-Dar, 2003). Though uncertain of their future, artists and viewers could revel in the comfort of community by "sharing a common fate, a singular desire: not to lose the human spirit" (Shen-Dar, 2003, p. 96).

Among the works of art created at Gurs which still exist today is a reproduction of an illustrated booklet that Trudl Besag made for a fellow inmate's 65th birthday (Slutsky & Weininger, 2016). On each page, a drawing that depicts the poor conditions in the camp is placed alongside a contrasting perspective of that scene through an idealistic depiction of it. As a birthday present, the booklet authenticated the desire of the prisoners to retain their humanity and consideration for each other. And as an archive, it attests to the resilience and optimism that gave inmates hope.

RAVENSBRÜCK

Located approximately 50 miles north of Berlin, Ravensbrück was the largest female concentration camp in Europe. The first transport of women arrived in May 1939, consisting mostly of German political prisoners (Saidel, 2001). Roughly 130,000 women were registered in the camp before its liberation in 1945 and conditions worsened significantly over the course of those six years (Morrison, 2000; Saidel, 2001). The women imprisoned there contended with starvation, unsanitary conditions and physical labor. They were also subjected to sexual exploitation and medical experiments. And yet the women at Ravensbrück developed an artistic culture within the confines of the camp. Morrison wrote:

> It is no small tribute to the human spirit that in the midst of all the exploitation and oppression, the suffering, even torture and death, women prisoners at Ravensbrück raised their sites above their circumstances and found the energy and vision to be creative (2000, p. 147).

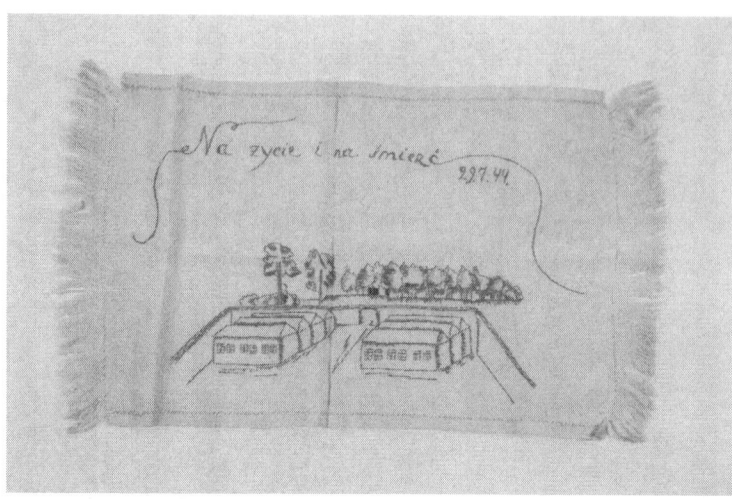

Figure 4.3 Embroidered doily made by a Polish inmate in Ravensbrück depicting the camp. Ravensbrück, 1944. Courtesy of the United States Holocaust Memorial Museum Collection, Gift of Bozenna M. Urbanowicz Gilbride.

These creative endeavors included poetry, singing and visual arts. The creative community at Ravensbrück existed under the threat of constant danger because the guards on duty there actively broke up and disorganized any group activity (Półtawska, 2018).

Taking a humorous tone, Czech dancer and costume designer Nina Jirsikova developed the *Ravensbrück Fashion Magazine*, illustrating ideas for how inmates could alter their uniforms to look more fashionable (Morrison, 2001). She drew her fellow prisoners as models, showing off their stark uniforms as if they were examples of high fashion. The secret magazine was passed around for amusement.

A number of craftworks from the Ravensbrück camp also exist, including jewelry, small toys and textiles. Prisoners in the camp routinely created gifts for each other—a phenomenon that Saidal (2001) noted was more common among female prisoners. On an embroidered doily (Figure 4.3) created by an unknown Polish inmate, the outline of a barracks is stitched in the center. The top reads: *Na zycie i na smierc* (*In life and death*). I was unable to obtain additional information on this specific piece, but suspect that the wording alludes to the communal struggle of the women imprisoned at the camp. In looking at the delicate stitching in the image, I am reminded of Leone's (2020) discussion of crafting as a tool for empowerment and community building. Leone wrote that: "given the social power of craft, when groups of people who are marginalized or oppressed gather together to craft, both process and product can become an awareness-raising tool and even a method of resistance to social and/or political oppression" (p. 10). Though she was not describing the craft community in Ravensbrück, her words are nonetheless applicable. Given the documentation of the close relationships that the women in the camp fostered, it is unlikely that this piece was created in isolation. Testimony has indicated that creating pieces of art and craft in the camp brought the women together in a cultural resistance against oppression (Saidel, 2001). The softness of materials used in the doily (Figure 4.3) serves to counter the harshness of the environment in which they were created. These items were likely intended as gifts to exchange between prisoners, but serve a secondary function as forces of resistance against dehumanization. In both functions, the art and craft items created in Ravensbrück represented avenues of community building within the camp.

AUSCHWITZ

The name *Auschwitz* is analogous with death, so it is surprising to learn of the extensive cultural activity that took place there. The Auschwitz-Birkenau State Museum holds thousands of pieces of art created by victims across the camp complex. The artistic impulse began with the first transports of Polish political prisoners who arrived in Auschwitz in June 1940. A number of skilled and celebrated artists were on these transports, and they "provided the starting impetus for artistic tradition in the camp" (Dalek & Swiebocka, 1989, p. 2). These transports of prisoners were stationed in carpenter and locksmith workshops; though in late 1940 and early 1941, these workshops were transferred and transformed into *Industriehof* where all craft workshops were located. Here, using the items at their disposal, prisoners such as Xawery Dunikowski and brothers Wladyslaw and Karol Kupiec began making their own pieces of art. This artistic tradition continued until the camp was liberated in January 1945. Surviving artist Janina Jaworska explained the need to create in Auschwitz:

> How did people sentenced to death have the time and will to care for cultural life in such circumstances? As a former prisoner in Auschwitz, I make the claim with all my determination that if there had been no such life at all, far fewer inmates would have survived the nightmare and lived to freedom (1975, p. 7).

A portion of the cultural activity at the Auschwitz complex occurred in Section BIIb of Auschwitz-Birkenau, the Terezín family camp (*Theresienstädter Familienlager* in German). To better contextualize the artistic activity in BIIb, I must first explain the family camp's inception. While most families sent to Auschwitz were immediately separated, the Terezín family camp was unique. In September 1943, over 46,000 Jews were deported to Auschwitz from the Terezín ghetto, in preparation for an inspection from the Red Cross. The Nazis were worried that Red Cross officials would ask for proof that the evacuated Jews were alive and in good health, so they established the family camp as an interim section. Two other transports from Terezín came in December 1943 and May 1944. Approximately 18,000 Jews from these transports were placed in the family camp, where they were given some privileges. They were allowed to keep their luggage and wear civilian clothing, and their heads were not shaved, though they were still tattooed with numbers. Their processing documents were coded, unbeknown to them, with an indication that they were to be gassed after six months. By July 1944, the family camp was liquidated. Some boys and men were assigned to work details, while the rest perished. Fewer than 1,500 survived.

During its brief existence, the children in the family camp lived under a false sense of comfort and security. Since they were not useful to work, the children were permitted to engage in educational and cultural activities. They were even given art materials by the German guards (Grant, 2002) who monitored the camp. A prominent Jewish leader in the Terezín ghetto, Czech Freddy Hirsh, was put in charge of the children's barracks within the family camp. Under his watch, children drew, played and even put on small performances. Surviving artist Marianne Grant taught painting techniques and nature study to the children in the family camp (Grant, 2002). Yehuda Bacon recalled drawing and dancing during the six months he spent in the family camp (Y. Bacon, personal communication, September 26, 2017).

In anticipation of a potential Red Cross visit, the guards asked artists in the family camp to paint murals for the children. Grant painted likenesses of beloved characters such as Bambi and Mickey Mouse, along with flowers, trees, and mushrooms (2002). Hirsh commissioned another artist, Dina Gottliebova, who had also been deported to Auschwitz from Terezín, to paint a mural in the children's barracks. She began painting a landscape scene; and when she noticed children nearby watching her, she asked them for input on what to paint in the barracks (Gottliebova, in Helstein, 2009). They requested Gottlibova paint a scene from the fairytale *Snow White and the Seven Dwarfs*.

Painting the mural of a fairytale scene was meaningful for both Gottlibova and the children. For the artist, the act of transforming the crude barracks wall into a canvas for Snow White gave her a sense of accomplishment and allowed her an opportunity to provide for the children in a way that only she could. Though she couldn't offer them extra rations of food or layers of clothing, she was able to remind them of a comforting, familiar, fantastical story which, as Haase (2000) stated, served as a "psychological defense" (p. 372).

Fairytale themes featured prominently in other artworks made in Auschwitz. Cards drawn by inmates in the Auschwitz construction office featured fairytale images. Having access to drawing tools and paper, workers in the construction office were known to trace images from a book that was found in 1943 (Dalek & Swiebocka, 1989), which they made into greeting cards and booklets to send to their children outside of the camp (Sieradzka, 2019). In his discussion of fairytale imagery in artwork by Holocaust survivors and second-generation survivors, Haase (2000) makes the point that this supported the use of imagination as a tool of liberation. Drawing the idealistic images into existence in the harsh world of Auschwitz was an attempt to liberate the mind from the surrounding atrocities. The metaphor of good triumphing over evil and adversity perhaps shed a glimmer of hope on the artists' situation.

The Auschwitz-Birkenau Museum also holds a number of albums created by prisoners in the camps. One album in particular was made by a group of male inmates, intended for a female group in the Budy sub-camp (Figure 4.4). The album is filled with personalized wishes for individual recipients, along with corresponding illustrations. Curators at the museum noted that this album, along with others, exemplifies how the inmates continued to care about the needs of others, despite their circumstances. An excerpt from the album reads:

> I wish that Hela joins Piotruś in holy matrimony as soon as possible
>
> May Emi return happily to Hamburg with Dad
>
> To Rachel, I wish that she takes Srulek for the long-awaited honeymoon
>
> May Hania return to her husband and children. (as cited in Sieradzka, 2019).

An especially odd phenomenon that was unique to Auschwitz was the development of the camp museum, which displayed inmate artwork. According to Dalek & Swiebocka (1989), the idea for a museum came about incidentally in 1941 when the camp commandant, Rudolf Hoss, caught prisoner Franciszek Targosz drawing a battle

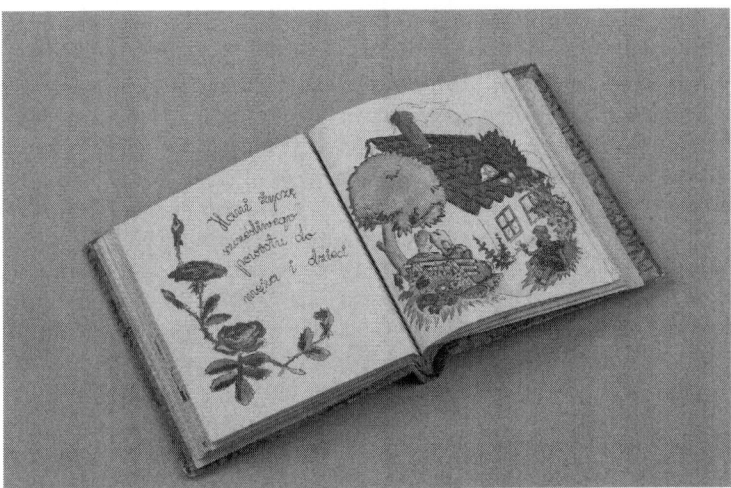

Figure 4.4 Artist Unknown. *Album from Budy Subcamp.* 1943–1944. From the collections of the Auschwitz-Birkenau State Museum.

scene that happened to include horses. Targosz evaded punishment because Hoss was a horse enthusiast, and was instead tasked with organizing the Lagermuseum. The museum displayed collections of items stolen from prisoners, as well as original artworks created by prisoners. The artwork on display had to be pleasurable to SS guards and the SS often commissioned pieces for the museum.

The museum became an entity of normality for imprisoned artists. More experienced artists offered instruction to beginners and an artistic community developed. Targosz even made space for artists to create their own work clandestinely and took strides to hide the works to avoid their makers getting caught. Artist Jan Baras recalled:

> I went to the museum from time to time after finishing work. This was due to my love for drawing but also because I wanted to meet others whose interests I could share. And then the possibility of drawing there, in the camp museum, enabled us to forget just for a moment the monstrous reality of the place. There was an atmosphere of freedom in the museum, and we created it ourselves (as cited in Dalek & Swiebocka, 1989, p. 10).

There is evidence of communal art making in camps and ghettos beyond the examples I have detailed. The lesser-known Banjica concentration camp, located in Belgrade, Serbia, was known to have an active creative community, which united prisoners of varying cultural backgrounds (Tomic et al, 2019). In Bergen-Belsen, a former designer gave art lessons to the children who had been on her transport from Budapest, using sticks and mud. (I will elaborate on this particular story in Chapter 6.) In addition to visual arts, captives in ghettos and camps engaged in other creative pursuits, including music, theater and writing (Karay, 1994; Seigelman, 1995; Tomic et al, 2019). For example, women held in the Skarżysko-Kamienna labor camp sang familiar songs together as a means of retaining their culture (Karay, 1994). The focus of this text is on the visual arts created in camps and ghettos, so it is beyond my scope to expound on the other cultural activities that occurred. However, the prominence of all the arts as a part of ghetto and camp life further supports the notion that creativity can build community, even in the bleakest of environments.

I want to clarify that art making, though abundant, was not a universal activity across Nazi systems. Such pursuits were dangerous and, for some, completely impossible to engage in. Of the 23,697 individuals registered at Banjica between 1941 and 1944 (Israeli, 2013), approximately 170 engaged in some type of visual art activity (Tomi et al, 2019), which is a rather small percentage. Still, these small numbers of artists had a major impact—on themselves, on their community, and on future viewers of their works. The desire to build a sense of community, foster relationships and recognize and care for the needs of others seemed to surpass the potential dangers inherent in communal art making. These efforts to create an artistic culture further emphasize the attempts by victims to retain a sense of normalcy and humanity.

COMMUNITY ART THERAPY PRACTICES

The artistic communities that developed in Nazi camps and ghettos bear similarities to contemporary community art therapy practices. Unlike clinical art therapy groups, which strive to ameliorate an individual's psychiatric symptoms, the goal of community art therapy groups is to support the needs of the community as a whole (Kapitan, et al., 2011; Nolan, 2019). Such groups often take place at inviting locations central to the community, with the aim of promoting in participants a sense of agency, connectedness and purpose (Nolan, 2019). The intent behind communal art making within camps and ghettos was to bolster the sense of humanity that had been taken away. The humanizing of marginalized populations—the act of building a collective voice for those who have been disempowered—is a critical function of community psychology and community art therapy.

Community psychology is an area informed by social justice practices. Community psychology aims to elevate the health of community members while remaining aware of the institutional, social and ecological factors that can impact a community (Duffy, 2019). In recent years, art therapists have recognized the need to move beyond the medical model to support health and wellbeing within traumatized communities. Morris and Willis-Rauch (2014) found that facets of the psychotherapy groups that are run in psychiatric units can be incongruent with art therapy values. In order to practice in accordance with social justice values, contemporary art therapists have broadened their work to include anti-oppressive practices, recognizing the systemic influences on communities that can result in suboptimal health conditions. With this, there has been an emergence of community art practices documented in art therapy literature (Klorer, 2014; Leone, 2020; Timm-Bottos, 2011; Ottemiller & Awais, 2016). Art therapists have developed community art groups in order to give voice to marginalized communities, develop bonds within the community, increase empathy and support growth and healing (Evans, Kivell, Haarlammert, Malhotra & Rosen, 2014; Ottemiller & Awais, 2016, Potash & Ho, 2011). By definition, community art therapy operates outside of a traditional psychiatric setting and takes place within a marginalized or traumatized community. Rooted in a social justice framework, community art therapy is not concerned with pathology, but instead promotes wellness and change at a communal level (Ottemiller & Awais, 2016).

The examples of communal art making in the ghettos, internment camps and concentration camps that I detailed in this chapter seem to embody the goals of community art therapy practices. Kapitan's (2009) recognition of the "emancipatory spirit of art against that which stifles and oppresses them in body, mind, and spirit" (p. 150) is applicable to the artistic communities that developed in captivity. The artists working within these environments were under extreme oppression, and yet were able to achieve a degree of healing through art making. The most comparable attributes of both community arts within the Holocaust and community art therapy practices are resistance and empowerment.

Art as Resistance

Dehumanization of prisoners was a critical component of the torture that endured in camps and ghettos. When asked why victims were dehumanized as part of the Nazis' Final Solution, former camp commander Franz Stangl simply explained that "it made it easier" (Berenbaum & Mais, 2009, p. 105). Degrading camp inmates was a way for guards to follow orders without questioning their own morals. By treating inmates as if they were less than human, adopting what Lifton (1986) referred to as "the Auschwitz self," Nazi perpetrators were able to torture and kill. The dehumanization of inmates became a crucial element in carrying out a mass genocide, and it occurred daily in every camp and ghetto. If we understand art making to be a human behavior (Dissanayake, 1995) or a humanizing pursuit (Gussak, 2019), then we can understand cultural activity as a means of bolstering the humanity that was disregarded by their captors.

The art of the Holocaust is often descried as a type of spiritual or cultural resistance (Moreh-Rosenberg, 2016; Blatter & Milton, 1981; Saidel, 2001). Langer (1996) challenged this idea of cultural resistance, arguing that an active cultural community, while perhaps beneficial, could not compete against the systematic genocide of the Holocaust. He also points out the challenge of viewing these artworks as anything other than manifestations of the tortuous environments in which they were created: "...we are asked to connect the humiliation of man, which is the subject of so many of these paintings, with an attitude that somehow transcends that humiliation" (1996, p. 53). This transcendence on the part of the viewer is difficult, especially since many of the images demand such a visceral response. However, we can view the images as attempts at cultural resistance by considering not only what they show, but also the efforts taken to create them. The engagement in art making, not just the art itself, was an act of cultural resistance. These artists, and other prisoners, were not equipped with the strength or power necessary to effectively fight their captors. Starvation, demoralization and lack of resources made it impossible for victims to overturn the power that was held over them. Known revolts, such as the Warsaw ghetto uprising, were ultimately unsuccessful and led to increased punishment and worsening conditions. Holocaust artists were unable to fully resist against their oppressors; however, they could reclaim some of the attributes that had been taken away from them. In building communities, sharing an appreciation for the arts and leaving a legacy, these artists staged a cultural resistance against dehumanization. Artistic pursuits intensified the will to live, afforded an increased sense of autonomy and reinforced a community (Karay, 1994), which allowed for a type of cultural rebellion. By creating, artists refused to submit to the oppression visited upon them. As Blattner and Milton (1981) explained: "They were rejecting the Holocaust's horrors even while they were drawing them" (p. 34).

These humanizing pursuits are not unlike those of art therapists working in community practices. Timm-Botos (2011) found that a community art therapy group could "realize the goal of relational transformation and meaningful action" (p.57). Community-based art therapy also promotes this transformation by providing an outlet for expression and self-discovery. This emboldens participants to appreciate themselves and resist the systematic inequities which oppress them. Community arts studios give individuals a space to redefine themselves, instead of internalizing the negative ways they are viewed by those who have more power, affluence or control. The act of self-expression in community art therapy groups can lead to a collective response of small transformations in participants and their societies (Timm-Botos, 2011).

Additionally, in making art and engaging with a community of fellow artists, individuals within the Holocaust were able to transcend their prisoner identity to take on that of artist. Affirming oneself as an artist added a characterization to their identity and contributed to an increased sense of purpose. Participation in communal art activities reinforced the artistic identity. Frederick Terna, who was inspired by the artists in the Terezín technical department, began to see himself as an artist while drawing in Terezín. This newfound identity led him to transcend his circumstances and envision a life for himself after the war. Artist Xawery Dunikowski was known to self-identify as an artist. According to fellow inmate Leon Turalski: "He drew portraits and considered it his present vocation" (Sieradzka, 2019).

Assuming the artist identity was a benefit that Morris and Willis-Rauch found in their community arts work, as participants "reframed themselves as artists within the microcosm of their group and within their communities" (2014, p. 28). In both historical and contemporary examples, the adoption of an artistic identity allows an oppressed individual to realize their own potential and resist the dehumanizing way in which others view them. By assuming an identity other than oppressed victim, artists build up the strength to fight systematic dehumanization. The commitment to their cause of resistance shows how individuals living under oppression can find meaning in the circumstance.

Empowerment

In a community art therapy practice, the art therapist strives to empower group participants who have been disempowered. The participants are viewed as agents of change through their artistic encounter (Morris & Willis-Rauch, 2014). Engagement in art making can be empowering, as it allows opportunities for choice and expression—luxuries that are often unavailable to many disenfranchised communities. Participants can choose the art materials they use, the way in which they use them and the content of their artistic creations (Kapitan, 2014). Additionally, the expression that comes out in the artwork can be a powerful form of communication and the realization that such emotions have been communicated can also foster empowerment (Kapitan, 2014; Morris & Willis-Rauch, 2014). Artistic expression can provide a voice to those who have been silenced.

The unique opportunity for self-expression may have also been an empowering experience for those creating in captivity. Art is often included in social activism as a symbolic representation of needs and as a way to communicate those needs to others

(Sharp, 1973). The artists who created collectively within camps and ghettos were well aware of each other's needs. They were living in the same environment and had to endure the same kind of suffering. However, having the ability to communicate their needs to the outside world—even to viewers of their artwork in the future— promoted empowerment. Artist testimonies indicate a need to document and share their reality, to negate Nazi propaganda and to tell the truth about what they endured (Blatner & Milton, 1981; Moreh Rosenberg, 2016). Although victim artists did not have the power to change their conditions or guarantee their own fates, they were able to communicate the truth. I am reminded of Potash and Ho's (2011) discussion of *satyagraha* (Gandhi, 1956), a term used to describe a force intended to promote truth. Promoting the truth allowed artists to educate future generations about the harsh realities they faced. Art making was a tangible way to communicate their truth in case they were unable to speak it.

Aside from the case of Friedl Dicker-Brandeis, communal art making in camps and ghettos did not require a formal leader or facilitator. The individual participants in such groups empowered each other through their drive to create. Empowerment arrived organically through the art-making process. As Jan Baras explained, artists working in the Auschwitz Museum created their own sense of freedom, which must have been an empowering experience. I think this came from the ability to change— however briefly—the tone of the environment from one that was menacing and dangerous to one that fostered creativity and community. Finding moments of beauty and collaboration ultimately bolstered the human spirit and led to empowerment, despite the efforts of the Nazis to crush that spirit.

Community Building

Potash and Ho (2011) noted that art making and art viewing can support participation in society. The individuals creating communally in captivity had been pushed out of their societies at the onset of Hitler's rise to power. Prior to their deportation to ghettos or camps, many were barred from attending school, working or visiting certain neighborhoods. As Nazi ideology took over, Jews and other groups were ousted from the societies they had once been integral parts of. Upon their arrival at the camps and at some of the ghettos, Holocaust victims were often separated from their families, leaving them alone in groups of unfamiliar people. There was a desperate need to feel like a part of a community, especially after years of marginalization. Art making allowed for that. Artistic communities became a familiar source of support and comfort. In fact, the bond among the Terezín artists was so close that after the war the lone survivor, Leo Haas, adopted fellow artist Bedrich Fritta's son, Tommy.

It is clear that communities were built through creative endeavors in the Holocaust. By crafting items for each other, as was common in Ravensbrück, or creating for outside parties, as in the instance of the Auschwitz album, victims fostered a lost sense of community. Forging a community was an act of resistance against the Nazi perpetrators who had cast victims out of their prior communities. As such, community building was itself empowering. Through communal creativity, victim artists were able to maintain and pass on the cultural and educational values that defined their pre-war lives (Karkay, 2014), as seen through the examples of Dicker-Brandeis and educators in the Auschwitz family camp. Artists were also able to celebrate birthdays and holidays, as in the example of Trudl Besag's birthday gift, highlighting

Dissanayke's example of art being used to "make special" (1995). They were also able to join together to create and share artwork, as seen in the Auschwitz Museum. Artists supported the artistic identities of their fellow artists and encouraged each other to keep working, even when some had lost the will to create. Indeed, communal art making in the Holocaust made it possible to achieve the social-action goals of stimulating empathy and fostering relationships (Potash and Ho, 2011).

Contemporary art therapists have the capacity to facilitate relationships and build community through the creative process (Potash and Ho, 2011). Although the examples from camps and ghettos that I shared in this chapter were not facilitated by art therapists, they exemplify how community art making can serve as a form of resistance, empower marginalized individuals and foster community building. These benefits rendered in Holocaust community arts examples are not dissimilar to the benefits we see in contemporary community art therapy practices. They also support the liberation psychology idea of uniting psyche and culture, "to witness pain as it issues from both quarters, and to enter the mess and fray of participation, solidarity, and responsibility" (Lorenz & Watkins, 2003, p. 20). By engaging in these artistic endeavors, the artists assumed great risk. However, their need to participate in a community, develop a sense of solidarity and assume a responsibility to promote the truth all seemed to outweigh the known risks. I hope that these historical examples can educate and support art therapists working in community settings and serve as a reminder of the power of an artistic community.

NOTE

1. This term, though dated, is used to stay consistent with the terminology used in testimony and related literature.

REFERENCES

Amishai-Maisels, Z. (1993). *Depiction and interpretation: The influence of the Holocaust on visual arts.* Tarrytown, NY: Pergamon Press.

Bak, S. (2001). *Painted in words.* Bloomington, IN: Indiana University Press.

Beinfeld, S. (2011). The cultural life of the Vilna Ghetto. In *Volume 1* (pp. 94–115). Berlin, New York: K. G. Saur. https://doi.org/10.1515/9783110968736.94

Berenbaum, M. & Mais, Y. (2009). *Memory and legacy: The Shoah narrative of the Illinois Holocaust Museum.* Lincolnwood, IL: Publications International, Ltd.

Blatner, J. & Milton, S. (1981). *Art of the Holocaust.* New York, NY: Routledge.

Costanza, M. (1982). *The living witness: Art in the concentration camps and ghettos.* New York, NY: The Free Press.

Dalek, J. & Swiebocka, T. (1989) *Suffering and hope: Artistic creations of the Oświęcim Prisoners* (J. Kosiec, trans.). Oświęcim, Poland: Panstwowe Muzeum Auschwitz-Birkenau.

Dissanayake, E. (1995). *Homo aestheticus: Where art comes from and why.* Seattle, WA: University of Washington Press.

Evans, S. D., Kivell, N., Haarlammert, M., Malhotra, K. & Rosen, A. (2014). Critical community practice: An introduction to the special section. *Journal for Social Action in Counseling & Psychology, 6*(1), 1–15.

Duffy, K. G. (2019). *Community psychology.* New York, NY: Routledge.

Dutlinger, A. D. (2001). *Art, music and education as strategies for survival: Theresienstadt, 1941–45.* New York, NY: Herodias.

Frankl, V. (1973). *The doctor and the soul. From psychotherapy to logotherapy.* New York, NY: Vintage Books.

Gandhi, M. K. (1956). Satyagraha in South Africa. In J. A. Jack (ed.). *The Gandhi reader: A source book of his life and writings.* New York, NY: Grove. (Original work published in 1928).

Grant, M. (2002). *I knew I was painting for my life: The Holocaust artworks of Marianne Grant.* Glasgow, Scotland: Glasgow Museums.

Green, G. (1978). *The artists of Terezin.* New York, NY: Hawthorn Books.

Gussak, D. (2019). *Art and art therapy with the imprisoned: Re-creating identity.* New York, NY: Routledge.

Haase, D. (2000). Children, war, and the imaginative space of fairy tales. *The Lion and the Unicorn, 24*(3), 360–377. doi:10.1353/uni.2000.0030

Helstein, H. (Director/writer/producer). (2008). *As seen through these eyes* (Motion Picture). United States: Parkchester Pictures.

Israeli, R. (2013). *The death camps of Croatia: Visions and revisions, 1941–1945.* New Brunswick, NJ: Transaction Publishers

Jaworska, J. (1975). Nie wszystek umrę... Twórczość plastyczna Polaków w hitlerowskich więzieniach i obozach koncentracyjnych 1939–1945. Warsaw, Poland: Książka i Wiedza.

Kantor, A. (1971). *The book of Alfred Kantor: An artist's journal of the Holocaust.* New York, NY: McGraw Hill.

Kapitan, L. (2014). Empowerment in art therapy: Whose point of view and determination? *Art Therapy, 31*(1), 2–3, doi: 10.1080/07421656.2014.876755

Kapitan, L., Litell. M. & Torres, A. (2011) Creative art therapy in a community's participatory research and social transformation. *Art Therapy, 28*(2), 64–73. doi:10.1080/07421656.2011.578238

Karay, F. (1994). The social and cultural life of the prisoners in the Jewish forced labor camp at Skarżysko-Kamienna. *Holocaust and genocide studies, 8*(1), 1–27.

Klorer, G. P. (2014) My story, your story, our stories: A community art-based research project. *Art Therapy, 31*(4), 146–154, doi: 10.1080/07421656.2015.963486

Langer, L. (1996). *Admitting the Holocaust: Collected essays.* New York, NY: Oxford University Press.

Leone, L. (Ed.). (2020). *Craft in art therapy: Diverse approaches to the transformative power of craft materials and methods.* New York, NY: Routledge.

Lifton, R. J. (1986). *The Nazi doctors: Medical killing and the psychology of genocide* (Vol. 64). New York, NY: Basic Books.

Lorenz, H. and Watkins, M. (2003). Depth psychology and colonialism: Individuation, seeing-through, and liberation. *Quadrant, 33,* 11–32.

Makarova, E. (2001). *Friedl Dicker-Brandeis.* Los Angeles, CA: Tallfellow/Ever Picture Press.

Milton, S. (2000). Culture under duress: Art and the Holocaust. In F. C. Decoste and B. Schwartz (Eds.). *The Holocaust's ghost: Writings on art, politics, law and education.* Edmonton, AB: University of Alberta Press, 84–96.

Moreh-Rosenberg, E. (2016). *The art from the Holocaust.* Cologne, Germany: Wienand Verlag.

Morris, F. J., and Willis-Rauch, M. (2014). Join the art club: Exploring social empowerment in art therapy. *Art Therapy, 31*(1), 28–36.

Morrison, J. G. (2000). *Ravensbrück: Everyday life in a women's concentration camp. 1939–45.* Princeton, NJ: Markus Wiener Publishers.

Nolan, E. (2019) Opening art therapy thresholds: Mechanisms that influence change in the community art therapy studio. *Art Therapy, 36*(2), 77–85, doi: 10.1080/07421656.2019.1618177.

Ottemiller, D. D. and Awais, Y. J. (2016). A model for art therapists in community-based practice. *Art Therapy*, *33*(3), 144–150.

Półtawska, W. (2018). Experimental operations at Ravensbrück concentration camp (T. Bałuk-Ulewiczowa, trans.). *Medical review – Auschwitz*. Originally published as "Operacje doświadczalne w obozie koncentracyjnym Ravensbrück." *Przegląd Lekarski – Oświęcim.* 1963: 90–97.

Potash, J. and Ho, R. (2011) Drawing involves caring: fostering relationship building through art therapy for social change. *Art Therapy*, *28*(2), 74–81, doi: 10.1080/07421656.2011.578040.

Rosenberg, P. (2001). *Learning about the Holocaust through art.* http://art.holocaust-education.net/.

Rosenberg, P. (2002). Mickey Mouse in Gurs: Humour, irony and criticism in works of art produced in the Gurs internment camp. *Rethinking History 6*(3), 273–292, doi: 10.1080/13642520210164508.

Saidel, R. G. (2001). *Women of Ravensbrück.* St. Petersburg, FL: Florida Holocaust Museum.

Seligman, Z. (1995). Trauma and drama: A lesson from the concentration camps. *The Arts in psychotherapy, 22*(2), 119–132. doi: 10.1016/0197-4556(95)00017-Y.

Sharp, G. (1973). The politics of nonviolent action. Boston, MA: Porter Sargent.

Shen-Dar, Y. (2003). Victory for the creative spirit behind barbed wire. In B. Gutterman & N. Morgenstern (eds.). *The Gurs Haggadah: Passover in perdition* (N. Kanner, Trans., pp. 95–101). Jerusalem, Israel: Devora.

Sieradzka, A. (2019). *Art at Auschwitz.* http://lekcja.auschwitz.org/en_18_sztuka/ Oświęcim: Państwowe Muzeum Auschwitz-Birkenau/Auschwitz-Birkenau State Museum

Slutsky, J. and Weininger, A. (eds.). (2016). *How it is but how it should be: Gurs in rhyme and sketch.* Skokie, IL: Illinois Holocaust Museum & Education Center.

Spenser, T. and Tarsi, A. (eds) (2001). *Art and medicine in Ghetto Theresienstadt: Drawings from the years 1942–1944.* [Exhibition catalogue]

Stein, L. (2013). *Beyond death and exile.* Cambridge, MA and London, England: Harvard University Press, https://doi.org/10.4159/harvard.9780674436299.

Timm-Bottos, J. (2011) Endangered threads: socially committed community art action. *Art Therapy*, *28*(2), 57–63, doi: 10.1080/07421656.2011.578234.

Tomić, I., Milić, V., Lazić, D. and Marinković, S. (2019). Psychological survival in Banjica concentration camp due to inmate creativity. A recommendation to future victims. *Austin Anthropology, 3*(2): 1008.

Trunk, I. (1972). *Judenrat: The Jewish Councils in Eastern Europe under Nazi Occupation.* New York, NY: The MacMillan Company.

Yad Vashem. *The Holocaust in France.* http://www.yadvashem.org/holocaust/france.

Yad Vashem. *The pen and the sword: Jewish artist and partisan Alexander Bogen.* http://www.yadvashem.org/yv/en/exhibitions/bogen/about.asp.

Yad Vashem. *Interview with Alexander Bogen, survivor and artist.* https://www.yadvashem.org/articles/interviews/alexander-bogen.html.

PART 2
RESEARCH

This part is an explication of my doctoral research examining the phenomenon of art making during the Holocaust. Chapter 5 is admittedly unconventional, as I use it to explain the motivation for my study and the steps I took in preparing and familiarizing myself with this work. I describe the research trips I took as a sort of active literature review to see artwork in person and meet with the curators and scholars who have studied this phenomenon. I also describe my criteria for recruiting participants and the decision to use a phenomenological research method. In Chapter 6, I introduce the reader to my participants by sharing their unique stories along with samples of their artwork. In Chapter 7, I detail the results of my study and explain the limitations that I faced in researching a phenomenon 75 years after it occurred.

* Chapters in this part have been adapted from Hlavek, E., (2020). A phenomenological inquiry into the art of the Holocaust. *Art Therapy*, *8*(3), 146–153.

https://doi.org/10.1080/07421656.2020.1780095

DOI: 10.4324/9781003160885-7

CHAPTER 5

ORGANIZING A STUDY OF HOLOCAUST ART

My introduction to the art of the Holocaust came at the end of a visit to the Terezín Memorial in November 2006. The memorial consists of a dozen sites in Terezín in the Czech Republic, where the Nazis forced 150,000 Jews into a walled-off ghetto and concentration camp, starting at the end of 1941. As the war closed out, Allied troops liberated Terezín in 1945.

The memorial, established in 1947, has preserved the barracks, work areas, crematoria and other facilities that the Nazis set up during the Holocaust in Terezín. Among them is the Small Fortress, which served as a Gestapo prison between 1940 and 1945. It is now a museum that houses several permanent exhibitions, including one that features Holocaust artwork created by child and adult prisoners at Terezín.

Going on this tour was incredibly informative, but also emotional and disturbing in a way I had not anticipated. Standing in the cramped rooms and walking along the railroad tracks that led the captive residents in and out of the ghetto made me think deeply about the day-to-day experience of those who had suffered in the ghetto. I could envision beleaguered travelers carrying pieces of the actual luggage that the museum displayed—across from the railroad tracks where I stood—having no idea what their futures held. I imagined them as prisoners crowding into an attic to secretly celebrate *Shabbat*, a tradition I had taken for granted.

Growing up in a strong Jewish community, I became aware of the Holocaust at an early age. The Jewish day school I attended through eighth grade displayed posters in the hallways each year to commemorate *Yom HaShoah*, Holocaust Remembrance Day. The posters revealed many historical facts about the Holocaust. However, their real impact came through the poignant images of prisoners and their surroundings, as photographed by the soldiers who liberated the camps.

I vividly remember photographs of corpses piled unceremoniously on a wagon and groups of emaciated men standing behind barbed wire. These haunting images underscored the mass scale of the Holocaust. The grainy black and white photographs made the individual victims and survivors difficult to distinguish, and the staggering statistics on the posters involved numbers too large to comprehend. I could only conceptualize the Holocaust as a large-scale genocide. However, that changed when I had the opportunity to tour Terezín. Walking through a single ghetto and learning what the residents had to contend with forced me to consider the Holocaust from a more individualistic perspective. In learning about the daily existence of prisoners in Terezín, I grasped a more personalized understanding of the Holocaust.

This sense of personalization grew when my tour group came to the museum's art collection. I saw hundreds of works created by both children and adults who were imprisoned at Terezín. Looking at the hundreds of images on display was a powerful experience. Although the works were small, they showed the Terezín experience through the eyes of these artists. Seeing them in totality, l was overwhelmed by the thought of the sheer number of people who had suffered in the very place where I stood. The next day, my group visited the Jewish Museum in Prague, where we saw even more artwork made by Czech Holocaust victims. The museum has 4,387 works

DOI: 10.4324/9781003160885-8

of art created by Jewish children in Terezín, most of them done under the guidance of Freidl Dicker-Brandeis.

When I reflected on the artworks I had seen at the Terezín Memorial and the Jewish Museum in Prague, I was struck by the extreme juxtaposition of their construction in one of the most destructive environments imaginable. How were the artists able to muster the will to create? I was about to start my graduate studies in art therapy, and implicitly felt there was a connection between the artwork I had just viewed and the career path I was about to embark on.

My visit to Terezín prompted me to write my master's thesis on Friedl Dicker-Brandeis's work with the children of Terezín. I also contemplated the idea of art making as a survival strategy. This led me to research other artists who had created art in the Nazi camps and ghettos, or while they were in hiding. I soon realized that the sum total of Holocaust artwork in the world is vast. Thousands of pieces were made by children and thousands more were created by adults in camps and ghettos across Europe. I continued to learn more about this phenomenon. My knowledge of Holocaust artwork expanded; and as I pursued my professional pathway in the art therapy field, I forged a route in which my art therapy identity became intertwined with the study of this genre of artwork.

When I began my doctoral studies in art therapy in 2015, I knew I wanted to further explore Holocaust artwork and the artists who created it. I felt certain that the study of Holocaust art could reveal benefits that we can also find in art therapy practices.

Each victim of the Holocaust who became involved in art making seemed to have a creative impulse that sparked an increased desire to live, not just exist. I wondered if art therapists could apply this mindset to support the needs of their clients.

And when I reviewed the scope of the literature on Holocaust artwork, it became apparent that few art therapists have examined or considered the collective body of this artwork in connection with their approach to art therapy practices. A significant gap exists in art therapy knowledge when it comes to understanding the nature and breadth of artwork created by Holocaust victims. Scholars in the fields of art history and cultural studies have certainly investigated Holocaust art; but only a minimal amount of literature in the art therapy sector addresses this body of artwork as a phenomenon.

Art therapy scholarship is limited to the study of specific artists to illustrate the function of witness in representing trauma (Leclerc, 2011); the legacy of Friedl Dicker-Brandeis (Kramer, 2000; Makarova, 1990, 2001; Wix, 2003, 2009); and Gussak's (2004) description of his experience viewing artwork at the Terezín memorial. I wanted to contribute further to this literature with testimony from actual surviving artists. I wanted to hear their stories firsthand to better understand why they chose to make art and learn about their experiences in doing so. I hoped then to apply what I learned from their experiences to art therapy theory and practice. These artists' works highlight the act of creativity as a life-giving response in the midst of a genocide. I wanted to speak directly with those who had chosen to engage creatively, some at the risk of their own life.

Many of the artists I have learned about did not survive the Holocaust. Some were murdered when their clandestine artwork was discovered (Green, 1978). Others, like the young prodigy Petr Ginz, perished before their talent could develop outside of captivity. Those who did survive are aging or have passed away. In developing my study, I recognized that I had a narrow window to meet and talk with the surviving artists. I wanted to capture the stories of these survivors firsthand, while they were still alive, to honor their experience and the tenacity of their very existence. Though they endured great suffering, I hoped to find continued meaning in their experiences by hearing their stories, learning from them and sharing them.

LIBERATION AND POST-LIBERATION ARTWORK

An immense collection of survivor artwork has been created since liberation (Amishai-Maisels, 1993; Presiado, 2012, 2015), which highlights the need that surviving artists harbor to continuously express and explore the impact of their experiences. Some artists continued to explore the theme of the Holocaust in their artwork decades after the war ended. Samuel Bak has spent his career integrating themes of Jewish history, personal history, destruction and rebuilding into his artwork through his use of symbols and metaphors. In a surrealistic style, Bak weaves his post-war life together with his Holocaust experience, resulting in colorful, allegorical oil paintings. Although he is far removed from the Holocaust, it remains present in his artwork 70 years after liberation.

During the years immediately following liberation, artists also responded to the Holocaust through their work. Picasso, for instance, began painting *The Charnel House* (on display at the Museum of Modern Art in New York) in 1944 after learning of the atrocities that occurred in the death camps. The artist used oils and charcoal to create a cubist painting that is reminiscent of his expression of the Spanish Civil War, *Guernica*. Inspired by newspaper images of corpses unceremoniously piled in camps, the painting is comprised of three lifeless figures laying in a tangle, their body parts dismembered and indistinguishable. The distorted faces evoke anguish and pain. Picasso limited his color palette to grays, giving the painting a somber tone. The artist's friend and cataloguer, Christian Zervos, stated that the painting represents "humanity, disgusting with murder, with hatred, chaos and affliction everywhere." He continued that Picasso's goal was "to show the terror of man at the sight of many corpses that weigh on his heart…" (as cited in Amishai-Maisels, 1993, p. 57).

The artworks made by survivors and second-generation survivors are certainly relevant to the field of art therapy, as they demonstrate how art making can support individuals in moving forward after a traumatic experience (Amishai-Maisels, 1993) or in responding to the burden of generational trauma. The artworks also allow survivors to more effectively convey the extent of their experience. Many survivors who created after the war used their artworks to communicate to others what had happened in ghettos and camps. In an interview with Yad Vashem, Yehuda Bacon explained: "It was a blessing that I could express everything I had experienced in my own language – I painted and wrote diaries" (Yad Vashem, 2021).

Artist Ella Liebermann-Shiber, who survived Auschwitz and a death march to the Neustadt camp, drew *Roll Call* (Figure 5.1) to explain to liberation troops what had happened (A. Bratman-Elhalel, personal communication, September 24, 2017) in the camps. The drawing depicts the array of horrors that the artist had seen during her captivity, including beatings and labor. Later in 1945, she began a series of drawings which she titled *On the Edge of the Abyss*, documenting the harrowing incidents

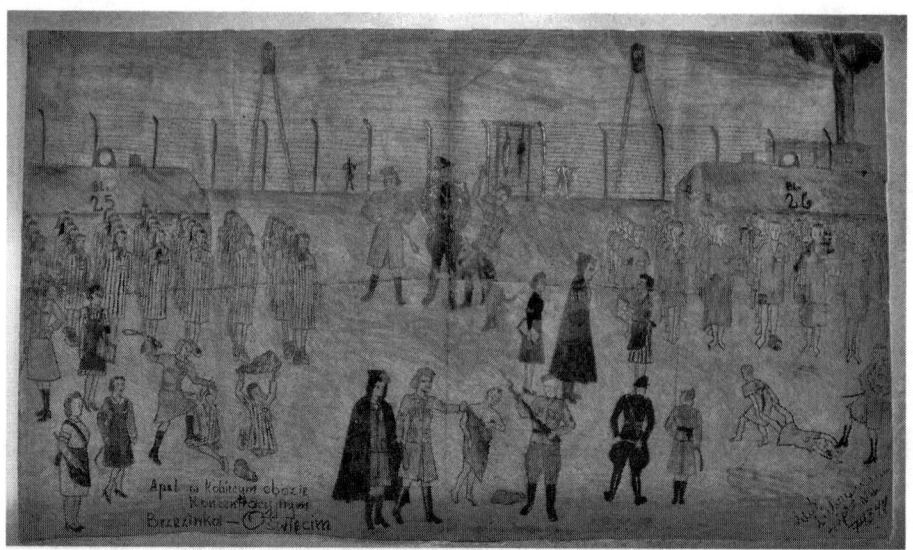

Figure 5.1 Ella Liebermann-Shiber (1927–1988). *Roll Call.* Neustadt camp, subcamp of Ravens-brück, 1945. Courtesy of the Ghetto Fighters' House Museum Art Collection, Western Galilee, Israel.

she witnessed throughout the war (Presiado, 2019). She was encouraged to draw by her husband, a Jewish officer in the Polish army whom she met at liberation. He thought that drawing such scenes would help release her of the trauma she had witnessed and experienced (Rosenberg, 2001). Liebermann-Shiber completed the series in 1948 and eventually donated it to the permanent collection of the Ghetto Fighters' Museum. The museum notes that the artist "regarded her dealing with these subjects in her artworks not only a documentation of harsh experiences and events, but also the beginning of a rehabilitative process" (Ghetto Fighter's House Archives, 2009).

In contrast to Samuel Bak, whose body of adult work encompasses Holocaust themes, and Liebermann-Shiber, who created a series of graphic drawings in the years following liberation, one artist I came across limited his post-liberation art to just one image related to the Holocaust. Auschwitz survivor Franz Reisz, who painted and drew during his captivity, made only a single post-liberation painting on the subject. In *Auschwitz* (Figure 5.2), Reisz painted a corpse lying in the dirt. In the background, he painted barracks and other buildings that are recognizable as part of the Auschwitz complex. The structures with smoke coming out and streaking across the painting are likely his depiction of the crematoria. A single bare tree and a dark, foreboding sky add to the desolate feel of the painting. According to Reisz's daughter, Sue Peyser, the artist poured his entire experience into this one piece and then moved on (personal communication, December 13, 2020). To her knowledge, he never revisited the theme of the Holocaust in any of his subsequent paintings. She did recall that *Auschwitz* hung in their dining room and she became accustomed to seeing it. Though the painting was prominently displayed in the family home, it was never discussed, which mirrored how her father acknowledged his Holocaust experience. He rarely spoke about his time in Auschwitz, though the ugliness of his experience was well known.

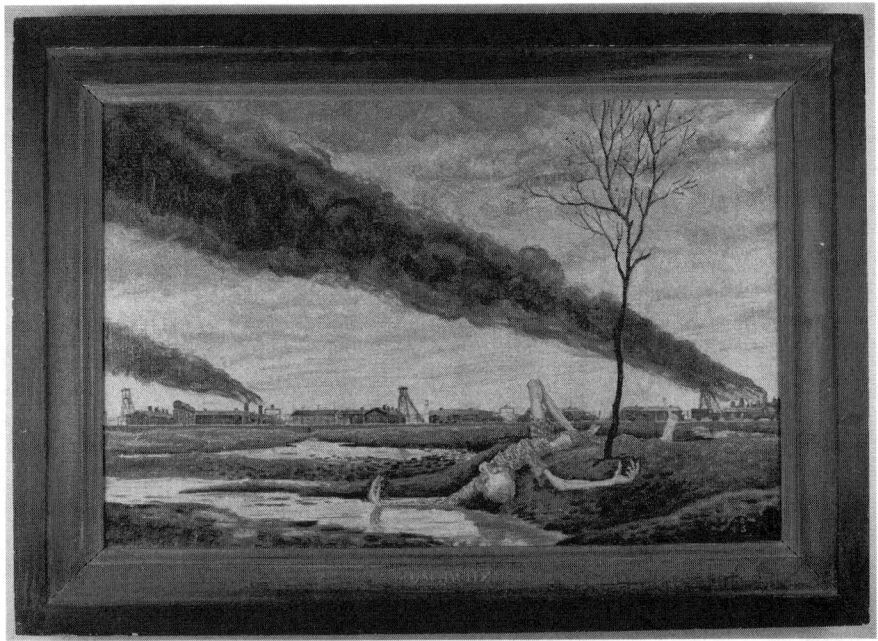

Figure 5.2 Franz Reisz (1909–1984). *Auschwitz. Auschwitz,* 1946. Courtesy of the United States Holocaust Memorial Museum Collection. Gift of Sue Peyser.

LIBERATION PERIOD ARTWORK

Although the examples of post-liberation Holocaust art are significant to the practice of art therapy, I chose to focus my research exclusively on artists who made artwork in a ghetto or camp system during the war. I began this inquiry intrigued by the artists who chose to create while in the midst of a genocide. The benefits of creating art in response to a traumatic experience are well documented in art therapy literature, though there is less exploration of the creation of artworks within an ongoing traumatic experience. The participants in this study, or the kin that they spoke about, had each created artwork while interned in camps or ghettos, or immediately after liberation while still ostensibly stuck in a camp or ghetto. This was the phenomenon of interest to me, so I limited my participants to artists who had created during the Holocaust.

Despite my decision to exclude artworks that were created years after liberation, I extended my criteria to include some artists who drew and painted immediately after liberation. I will call this *liberation period artwork,* as post-liberation art encompasses works made in studios and homes geographically and psychologically distant from the camps and ghettos. The artworks made in the liberation period remained close to the Holocaust and are therefore more connected to the body of Holocaust artwork I have discussed in this text. There are two main reasons for this. First, many artists who created during the Holocaust also created in the post-liberation period, including two of my eventual participants, Halina Olomucki and Yehuda Bacon. Much of the artwork made by artists during and immediately after captivity is stylistically similar and, as Presiado (2016) found, shares an artistic language. It is therefore impossible to understand and discuss the experience of a Holocaust artist without including all works that they may have made in the environments of the Holocaust. Liberation period works were created by artists who remained in a ghetto or camp in the days and weeks after the liberation troops arrived. These artists had limited materials to work with, just as before liberation, and remained in poor health. They were still surrounded by death and despair; and, with more freedom to roam camp grounds, they ultimately discovered even more evidence of destruction. They were also still in a state of shock and unable to fully trust that they were finally free. As documents, the liberation period artworks are equally authentic, as the artists' memories of events were fresh. Drawing about their captivity in the exact places they were held captive assisted the artists in recalling specific events that they had witnessed.

It is also important to understand that the experience of liberation was not the joyous occasion that we often assume it was. Survivor testimony indicates that while liberation was ultimately a pivotal moment and provided an initial sense of relief, the weeks and months that followed were a period of confusion, fear and terror. Zapruder (2002) quoted Alisa Ehrmann Shek's diary entry from the days after the Terezín ghetto was liberated: "Here and there a bent over figure drags himself from barracks to barracks.... almost everyone has died. Only a few are still groaning, whimpering, and sobbing. And peace is breaking over this field of death" (p. 402). Although victims were free from Nazi persecution after US, British and Soviet forces liberated them, their lives were shattered. Many were ill and in mourning for those who had not made it to liberation. Having lost family and friends, these survivors had no place to go and no sense of how the world outside had been ravaged by the war. Many victims were brought to displaced persons camps, where they were fed and given medical treatment; but in these camps they also became aware of the extent of the damage that had occurred. In testimony for the Midwest Center for Holocaust Education, Judy Jacobs explained the contradiction of liberation: "Well, it was, it was a relief but of course that's when all the bad information subsequently came, so it was a short-lived feeling of jubilation" (1999, p. 18). Liberation was an uncertain time and marked the beginning of survivors' attempts to reconstruct their lives. For these reasons, my study includes the experience of creating within a camp or ghetto in the aftermath of liberation.

PARTICIPANTS

I initially began this study as part of my doctoral research in 2017 and was able to interview additional survivors and second-generation survivors for this text. My options for possible participants were confined to those who had survived and remained alive and in good health. Because I was asking participants to discuss an egregiously painful portion of their life, I had to select participants who would be comfortable sharing these experiences. Some survivors, like Reisz, prefer not to talk about their experience in the Holocaust. Other survivors feel it is important to share their stories, but do so without emotion, in an attempt to keep the past behind them (Israeli, Regev & Goldner, 2021). The effects of aging on survivors' cognitive and physical abilities, as well as their apprehension about sharing their stories in one-to-one interviews, further narrowed my possibilities for participants. While setting up this study, a colleague sent me an article from the *Jewish Journal* on Kalman Aron, a Holocaust survivor who had drawn during his internment in the Riga ghetto and forced labor camps (Arom, 2017). I emailed the journalist who wrote the article in an attempt to connect with Aron. The journalist graciously tried, but Aron's health had unfortunately declined and he was unable to participate in my study. He passed away a year later. I recognized that the age of my potential participants was a limiting factor.

Given these requirements, I selected my participants as a convenience sample. I began by contacting Hilary Helstein, the director and producer of the 2009 documentary *As Seen Through These Eyes*, which featured six Holocaust artists. Since the film was less than a decade old, I anticipated that some of the artists in it were still alive and in good health. Helstein kindly provided me with contact information for a few of the individuals she interviewed, including Yehuda Bacon, Samuel Bak and Frederick Terna. I also reached out to an art therapist, Sherri Jacobs, who works with Holocaust survivors in Kansas City. Though none of her clients created art during their internment, she shared that her mother-in-law is a survivor who, guided by her mother, participated in spontaneous art lessons while interned in Bergen-Belsen. Ms. Jacobs put me in touch with her mother-in-law, Judy Gondos-Jacobs, who agreed to be interviewed.

SECOND-GENERATION SOURCES

Through my literature review, I came across artwork by Halina Olumucki which I found especially poignant. Olomucki drew regularly throughout her internment in the Warsaw ghetto and Birkenau, as well as after liberation. Sujo (2001) noted the consistency in Olomucki's style across her body of work. Her drawings are almost all figurative, with careful attention paid to the expression on each figure's face. The images are laden with anguish and fear, and tenderly convey the emotion of the artist's experience. Olomucki's works have been heavily discussed in Holocaust art literature (Blatter and Milton, 1981; Costanza, 1982; Presiado, 2016; Sujo, 2001) and I desperately wanted to learn more. I contacted the art museum complex at Yad Vashem, the world Holocaust museum in Jerusalem, to locate Olumucki. I was told that she had passed away in 2007, but I was able to obtain contact information for her daughter, Miriam Alon. Though not a survivor herself, Alon has written about and presented on her mother, and was able to serve as a secondary source of information. I was eager to know more about Olomucki's artwork, so I expanded my criteria again to include the children of Holocaust artists. I knew that this broader view would allow me to learn about more artists. I wanted to collect as much information about Holocaust artists as possible and realized that I might only be able to do so from second-generation survivors.

The unique psychology of second-generation survivors has been studied by American and Israeli researchers (Epstein, 1988; Harris, 2020; Levitt, 2007) interested in the transmission of intergenerational trauma. Harris (2020) noted that "as the Holocaust itself moves further into history, it remains a present fact for many children of survivors still mediating their own families' relationships and psychological postures" (p. 72). Although second-generation survivors did not experience the Holocaust firsthand, their connection to it runs deep. When I interviewed Alon, she admitted that she did not realize how common the burden of intergenerational trauma was to second-generation survivors. She described hearing another child of survivors speak on Holocaust Remembrance Day a decade prior and the subsequent relief she felt that "It's not just me" (M. Alon, personal communication, September 25, 2017). For most of her life, Alon had felt the burden of her parents' Holocaust experience (both Halina Olomucki and her husband were survivors), which was incongruent with the safe life she was raised in. This seems to be true of other children of survivors, who grew up in the shadow of the Holocaust's memory. Levitt (2007) found that second-generation survivors experienced an identification with their parents and lost ancestors, as so much of the way they were parented was impacted by the Holocaust experience. The legacy of the Holocaust is often intertwined with their own life experiences (Harris, 2020). To make sense of it, many second-generation survivors strive to reconstruct their parents' stories to reconcile the past with the present and confront the realities their ancestors faced (Blum, 2007). The curiosity that many children of survivors have, as well as the burden of intergenerational trauma, made Alon and other second-generation survivors useful participants in my study. By recalling what their parents had shared with them over time, combined with her own memories of their parents' attitudes, they could reconstruct a sense of their parents' Holocaust experience. This was also aided by factual information from archival sources housed in museums.

In preparation for this text, I set out to find more artists, or kin of artists, to interview. I contacted the curators I had met at Yad Vashem, Beit Terezín and the United States Holocaust Museum and Memorial for suggestions, and was fortunate enough to be put in touch with additional artists and family members of deceased artists. I completed a second phase of my study using the narrative accounts of Helga Hošková-Weissová; Thomas Geve and his daughter Yifat; and the daughter and niece of the late Alisa Ehrmann Shek.

RESEARCH METHODOLOGY

When I began to review the literature on the art of the Holocaust, I soon learned how common art making had been. These creative endeavors were pursued in a wide range of camps and ghettos across Europe. The recognition that artwork was made in Polish ghettos, French internment camps, German concentration camps, and Serbian labor camps led me to conceptualize the topic of Holocaust artwork as a phenomenon. Holocaust scholar Blattner also viewed this topic as a phenomenon (1981). After labeling my research interest as such, I decided a phenomenological research method would be most fitting.

Phenomenology is credited to Edmund Husserl, who sought to examine experiences outside of psychological and naturalist methods (Zahavi, 2003). Husserl's writings suggest that he viewed phenomenological research as an adventure in which he could immerse himself. His philosophy emphasized the use of *epoché*, a perspective from which previous judgments and assumptions are suspended in order to fully engage with the phenomenon. This became a critical approach for me in collecting and analyzing my data, considering that general information on Holocaust camps and ghettos contradicts any notions of creativity and beauty. The intent of phenomenological inquiry is to "explicate the essence, structure or form" (Kirby, 2016, p. 23) of a lived experience. Phenomenological researchers search underneath the surface of a narrative to extrapolate and decipher a meaning structure of what is occurring, or has occurred, in a given situation (Giorgi, 2009). While the artwork I had observed was striking, I found myself most interested in the individuals who created it and what motivated them to take on such a risky and complicated endeavor, making their art in such dire living conditions. Since phenomenological research is a study of "human experiential and behavioral phenomena" (Giorgi, 2012, p. 4) in a scientific, but not reductionist manner, this methodology was an appropriate choice.

I decided to apply Giorgi's descriptive phenomenological method since I was a novice researcher. In this system, Giorgi establishes a specific protocol for collecting and analyzing data. I could appreciate his step-by-step approach for my own phenomenological inquiry—a process that I will elaborate on in Chapter 7. I was also attracted to Giorgi's descriptive method because it is a system that allows phenomenology to inform psychology. Building on Sartre's (1956) belief that a phenomenological philosophy can support psychology more deeply and accurately than positivistic or empirical research, Giorgi strived to establish a synergy between phenomenology and psychology. This aligned with my own hypothesis that the phenomenon of Holocaust art could inform my art therapy practice. My hope was that by understanding the psychological benefits derived from this phenomenon, I could guide my clients to achieve similar benefits in their own art-making process.

RESEARCH GOALS

To delve into the lived experience of these artists, I organized a phenomenological inquiry into the experience of art making during the Holocaust. The inquiry had two goals: to honor these artists by sharing their stories and helping their legacies live on; and to uncover how art making supported them in the face of extreme adversity. This latter goal would also help me to guide my art therapy clients as they navigate their own struggles.

I wanted to change the way art therapists look at Holocaust artwork by shifting the focus from the perspective of a guide, such as Dicker-Brandeis, to that of the participants: the victims who took it upon themselves to create. I did not intend to draw implications for the treatment of PTSD and the benefits of art therapy in resolving a traumatic experience, which are already well documented in art therapy literature. The motivation to create after a genocide is obvious: there is a desperate need to process and reconcile the experience once an individual knows they are safe and free. I was curious, though, as to why artists took severe risks to make art in the midst of a genocide when they knew the inherent dangers. For camp and ghetto prisoners, daily life was traumatic; yet they managed to wedge opportunities into their days and nights to create works of art despite the ongoing streams of horror and fear that permeated their existence. Because Holocaust artwork was created during extended life-threatening situations, it provides what Jankevičiūtė referred to as "authentic evidence" (G. Jankevičiūtė, personal communication, March 31, 2016) of the victims' experience. The artwork is raw and reflects a sense of urgency and fragility that is intensified by the chronicity of such events. This evidence is in the form of the victims' experience, created in the midst of living through it.

An inquiry into the organic, self-motivated example of art making offered a unique—and quickly dwindling—opportunity to understand the perspective of the artists. That victims made art while fully aware of the inherent risks suggests that the benefits outweighed the dangers. By examining the process of art making in the Holocaust, I hoped to discern how victims potentially benefited and what purposes their creative endeavors served. I strived to understand the essence of the phenomenon of creating art in camps and ghettos, and began by asking the artists to tell me about their experience making art during the Holocaust. I hoped that understanding their experience and how it affected them would lead me to better recognize what my clients might get out of the creative process.

BIASES AND ETHICAL CONSIDERATIONS

In developing my study, I was keenly aware of the biases I possessed and the ethical considerations that are present with such a sensitive topic. I know that I have a significant cultural bias in this research. As a Jewish woman raised in a strong Jewish community, I always recognized the relevance of the Holocaust. Although I have no direct connection to victims, as my ancestors all immigrated to the United States prior to WWI, there is a cultural impact that I cannot deny. The burden of the Holocaust is something that I suspect all Jewish people experience on some level. To imagine living in Europe during Hitler's reign is a terrifying thought. I was acutely aware of this as I freely roamed the streets of Berlin in 2016 and considered how lucky I was to live in the time and place that I do. As a Jewish artist, I find that this research resonates with me on various fronts of my life. This resonance has served as a motivator and increased my passion and enthusiasm toward the study. However, it also presents a significant bias.

The study of Holocaust artwork brings up a number of ethical dilemmas. The serious nature of the subject cannot be handled lightly. Because I am so familiar with the work, I am less shocked by its disturbing nature. I continue to find the work upsetting and intense, but I am prepared for that reaction. I recognize that as a researcher, I need to prioritize sensitivity and respect toward those who have agreed to share their stories (Finlay, 2011). I am aware that I need to approach this topic with the utmost care to show respect for the victims and demonstrate my genuine interest and investment.

I did not want my participants to require anonymity, since it was important for me to be able to write about and discuss the specific individual in order to honor their experience. I wanted to present my participants as dignified human beings with their own distinguishing histories and attributes beyond those of surviving artists. Fortunately, each of the individuals I interviewed requested that their names be used. For many of them, telling their story is "the call, a responsibility to speak" (Y. Bacon, personal communication, September 26, 2017).

RESEARCH TRIPS

Berlin

I was fortunate enough to make two overseas research trips during my doctoral studies to deepen my familiarity with this body of artwork. Both trips came about suddenly, but they ultimately provided me with invaluable data. My first trip was to Berlin in the spring of 2016 to see the German Historical Museum's groundbreaking exhibit, co-curated by Eliad Moreh-Rosenberg of Yad Vashem's art museum and Walter Smerling of the German Foundation for Art and Culture. *Art from the Holocaust* featured 100 works of Holocaust artwork from the Yad Vashem collection. This was the largest exhibit of such works to be displayed outside the museum's archives in Jerusalem. Then-Chancellor Angela Merkel opened the exhibit on January 25 and it ran through April 3. The fact that these works were being displayed in the capital of Germany, where Hitler's reign began in 1933, was a testament to progress and education. Additionally, the collaboration between an Israeli and German organization underscored the appreciation for this type of education.

At the time, I had not seen a large collection of Holocaust artwork since my trip to Prague. I had viewed individual pieces or small collections on display at the U.S. Holocaust Museum and the Illinois Holocaust Museum and Education Center; but I had not been able to view a vast collection since beginning my research a decade earlier. I wanted the opportunity to see the artwork curated in the manner I was researching it: in other words, I wanted to see an exhibit of this scope spanning multiple camps, ghettos and artists. I anticipated that viewing the art as one collection, instead of organized by artist or location, would further help me to conceptualize this body of artwork as a phenomenon.

The museum was also hosting a series of lectures to accompany the exhibit. Once I had booked my travel, I identified a lecture that was to be delivered in English during the week I would be in Berlin. Dr. Giedrė Jankevičiūtė, an art historian at the Vilnius Academy of Arts in Lithuania, would present the lecture. I emailed Dr. Jankevičiūtė ahead of time and asked if she would be willing to meet with me to talk more about her research. She responded by suggesting that we meet after her lecture to schedule a time to talk the following day.

I spent my first full day in Berlin immersing myself in the subject of Holocaust art. I started with a visit to the Berlin Jewish Museum. As the largest Jewish museum in Europe, it walks the viewer through the history of the German Jewish people, starting with the Middle Ages. Though I was familiar with the history, it was still jarring to see how comfortable German Jews had been within the larger community and how quickly they were disenfranchised. One particular part of the exhibit showed pictures of Jews who had fought in the German army in WWI, highlighting how strong their German identity had been. And yet there were photographs of Nazis desecrating the graves of these German-Jewish soldiers.

The museum did not house art made in any German camps, though there were installations and exhibits created in response to the Holocaust. One particularly poignant exhibit was a collection of artworks by Russian Holocaust survivor Boris Lurie. After surviving four years in German camp Buchenwald, Lurie immigrated to New York to study art. He was shocked that the art world was not responding to the atrocities of the Holocaust and in 1959, he founded the NO!art movement with two other artists. The movement served as a counterforce to the trendy abstract impressionism and pop art movements. Using mixed media, Lurie aimed to bring "real life" to the forefront of art, believing that it is the artist's responsibility to tell the reality of the world. The following quote was displayed on a panel above his artwork: "You ask if artists should be responsible world citizens. I definitely think they should... I think the artist ought to try to be no different from any other mortal in this respect" (1962).

Lurie's most controversial image was *Railroad Collage*, in which he collaged a photo of a pinup model over the image of corpses in an extermination camp. His commentary was not subtle; but after enduring a camp, he was adamant that the world should know about the extent of the damage and reconsider their priorities. Another quote by Lurie, from an early exhibit in 1961, is etched into the wall entering his exhibit at the Jewish Museum. It reads:

> Welcome to this exhibition. If your eyes and mind serve you well, you will see something new. You will find no secret languages here, no fancy escapes, no hushed, muted silences, no messages beamed at exclusive audiences. Art is a tool of influence and urging. We want to talk, to shout, so that everybody can understand. Our only master is our truth (Involvement Show, 1961).

Lurie's words and mission set the tone for the rest of the afternoon. I felt a new surge of motivation for my research and saw how it fitted with the increasing social justice emphasis in art therapy theory and practice.

I visited the *Art of the Holocaust* exhibit in the afternoon. The room it was displayed in was understated and did not have the same feel as the dark, gray room that housed Lurie's exhibit or the intentional dim lighting at the US museum. It was clear that the curators intended for the art to speak for itself. The images ranged from hopeful to grotesque. Their small size required viewers to get close to them in order to absorb the details. Though they were displayed in simple frames, many of the pieces showed wear, indicating the challenge it took for the artist to preserve them. I thought about Lurie's statement and how this artwork served as the collective voice of Holocaust victims. Through these small pieces, they found a way to shout.

I spent three hours in the exhibit. After looking at each of the 100 pieces, I sat in an alcove where I could read quotes from the artists that were projected on the walls. Then I returned to the pieces, to view them again in the context of the artists' words. When it was time, I walked to a small auditorium to hear Dr. Jankevičiūtė speak. She discussed the artworks created in the ghettos in Lithuania by Alexander Bogen, Esther Lurie and Jacob Lipchitz. I was grateful to learn more about the pre-war lives of those artists and about their individual approaches for creating art within the ghettos. Dr. Jankevičiūtė also spoke about the rise of anti-Semitism in Lithuania during WWII, despite the presence of large Jewish communities there. We spoke briefly after her lecture and agreed to meet for breakfast the next morning.

Holocaust artwork is a niche topic and I valued any opportunities for discourse on the subject. I was grateful to meet with Dr. Jankevičiūtė and hear her perspective as a contemporary art historian. Dr. Jankevičiūtė described the artwork from the Holocaust as *authentic evidence*—a term that has stuck with me throughout my research process. I think her use of the word *authentic* has double meaning. It is authentic in the way that evidence must be: it comes as direct testimony from those who experienced the Holocaust. It is not evidence found by an outside party, but authentic—or true to its origins. There is also an emotional connotation of the word *authentic*, suggesting that this artwork tells us not only what happened, but how the artists experienced the events depicted in their art. The details come directly from the artists, who sought to authentically depict their experiences in the moment they were happening. I have since conceptualized the artwork of my clients as *authentic evidence*. The artwork created in art therapy sessions is evidence of a struggle or hardship, and also of the subjective feelings of living through such an experience and the emotions it evokes.

Israel

After my trip to Berlin, I felt reconnected with the art of the Holocaust. I completed my literature review and began setting up my course of study. I had considerable enthusiasm for this research and was eager to dive in. In the summer of 2017, I began making plans to interview each artist. It was easy to schedule a meeting with Frederick Terna at his home in Brooklyn, just a few blocks from where I had started my career at the Pratt Institute. I knew that the other participants would not be as accessible. Then one morning, I unexpectedly found a drastically discounted flight to Tel Aviv from Washington, D.C. and was able to travel to Israel in late September. I quickly set up interviews with Yehuda Bacon and Miriam Alon, and also arranged research visits to the Yad Vashem Art Museum, the Ghetto Fighters' Museum, and Beit Terezín, an Israeli organization established on Kibbutz Givat Hayim in 1975 to commemorate the Jews of Terezín. A family friend hosted me for a few nights in Tel Aviv and graciously drove me to Beit Terezín and the Ghetto Fighters' Museum. I met with curators at each location and was able to see the artwork on exhibit, in addition to other pieces in the museum archives.

The trip was a whirlwind. In under a week, I visited four cities and three museums, and interviewed two participants. I spent a night with Russian-Israeli art therapist Elena Marakova, who has written extensively on Friedl Dicker-Brandeis. We talked about the art of the Holocaust as it pertains to art therapy and the continued meaning that is found by sharing it with others for educational and therapeutic purposes. At Beit Terezín, I saw a collection of original artworks from Leo Hass, Otto Ungar, Bedrich Fritta, and Karel Fleishmann, all of whom I wrote about in my literature review. I also got to see the original book *Tommy*, which Fritta had made for his son's third birthday in Terezín. At the Ghetto Fighters' Museum, I saw the tiny drawings that Joseph Richter made on newspaper in transit to the Sobibor camp and a fragmented drawing by Joseph Bau, which curators had reconstructed like a puzzle. Though there were still pieces missing, the drawing showed a group of men in prisoner uniforms carefully dividing a loaf of bread to share.

I had previously toured the main exhibits at Yad Vashem, but this was my first time visiting the art museum there. Yad Vashem holds 10,000 artworks from the Holocaust, though only a fraction of the collection is on display at any given time. I spoke briefly with Eliad Moreh-Rosenberg, the chief curator, who had curated the exhibit in Berlin. I also spoke at length with Liat Shiber, who walked me through the artwork on display and shared literature from their archival collection. I was grateful to converse with the leading experts in the field of Holocaust art and to be able to look directly at an image while discussing the artist who created it. After exhausting the resources at the art museum, I went into the main museum to listen to recorded testimony from some of the artists whose work I had just seen, including Halina Olomucki and Alexander Bogen.

CONCLUSIONS

This chapter may have been unconventional, but I wanted to share with readers the motivators that led me to this research and the ways in which I immersed myself in it. Seeing the artwork in person, visiting the places where the artists actually made this artwork and learning about the series of events that preceded the establishment of ghettos and camps all helped me to contextualize this research. I wanted to get as close as possible to it and to understand the onset of the phenomenon as best I could. And as close as I got, I know there is still more to learn, to understand and to uncover. Frankl (1973) suggested that it is impossible for anyone to fully understand the experience of the Holocaust. Outside researchers, by definition, lack a first-hand perspective and therefore cannot empathize with or even fathom the series of events that occurred. On the contrary, those who survived the Holocaust are unable to distance themselves from it. Their accounts are hardened by their time as prisoners. Additionally, the deformed reality of one's time in a camp or ghetto can seem distorted, as the experiences challenge the conventions that outsiders would assume. As Frankl noted, "the standard measurement applied to the deformed lives was itself deformed" (1973, p. 93). Outside researchers, as would be expected, can never totally absorb the experiences that those who were imprisoned in the ghettos and camps suffered through.

To this end, researchers have developed theories based on consistencies that exist within the recollections of survivors. I suppose my process of understanding Holocaust art is similar. Although I have spent time with surviving artists, viewed collections of the artworks and read the appropriate literature, there is still an unfillable gap in my knowledge. The research and results presented in this text are simply an accumulation of how I have come to comprehend this phenomenon as an outsider. I found consistencies between sources and developed my theories based on thematic reoccurrences. My findings are ultimately tainted with my own biases, as well as the biases of my sources. That is the reality of historical research: there are inherent limitations. While I argue in support of my findings, I am aware that other theories and conclusions may also exist. I have written this chapter in order to show how I approached this research topic and ultimately arrived at the findings that will be discussed in Chapter 7. The remainder of this section presents relevant details concerning my phenomenological study.

REFERENCES

Amishai-Maisels, Z. (1993). *Depiction and interpretation: The influence of the Holocaust on visual arts.* Tarrytown, NY: Pergamon Press.

Arom, E. (2017). Saved by art: How one man's skill got him through seven Nazi camps and the difficult years that followed. *Jewish Journal.* https://jewishjournal.com/

Blatner, J. & Milton, S. (1981). *Art of the Holocaust.* New York, NY: Routledge.

Blum, H. P. (2007). Holocaust trauma reconstructed: Individual, familial, and social trauma. *Psychoanalytic Psychology, 24*(1), 63–73.

Costanza, M. (1982). *The living witness: Art in the concentration camps and ghettos.* New York, NY: The Free Press.

Epstein, H. (1988). *Children of the Holocaust: Conversations with sons and daughters of survivors.* New York, NY: Penguin Group USA.

Finlay, L. (2011). *Phenomenology for therapists: Researching the lived world.* Hoboken, NJ: John Wiley and Sons.

Frankl, V. (1973). *The doctor and the soul. From psychotherapy to logotherapy.* New York, NY: Vintage Books.

Giorgi, A. & Giorgi, B. (2003). The descriptive phenomenological psychological method. In P. M. Camic, J. E. Rhodes and L. Yardley (eds.). *Qualitative research in psychology: Expanding perspectives in methodology and design.* Washington, DC: American Psychological Association, pp. 243–273.

Giorgi A. (2009). *The descriptive phenomenological method in psychology: A modified Husserlian approach.* Pittsburgh, PA: Duquesne University Press.

Giorgi, A. (2012). The descriptive phenomenological psychological method. *Journal of Phenomenological Psychology, 43*(1), 3–12.

Green, G. (1978). *The artists of Terezin.* New York, NY: Hawthorn Books.

Gussak, D. (2004). Art made it real: My Terezín musings. *Journal of Cultural Research in Art Education, 2004*(22), 155–161.

Harris, J. (2020). An inheritance of terror: postmemory and transgenerational transmission of trauma in second generation Jews after the holocaust. *The American Journal of Psychoanalysis, 80*(1), 69–84.

Helstein, H. (Director/writer/producer). (2008). *As seen through these eyes* (Motion Picture). United States: Parkchester Pictures.

Israeli, R., Regev, D. & Goldner, L. (2021). The meaning, challenges, and characteristics of art therapy for older Holocaust survivors. *The Arts in Psychotherapy, 74,* 101783.

Kirby, J. K. (2016). An existential-phenomenological investigation of women's experience of becoming less obsessed with their bodily appearance. *Indo-Pacific Journal of Phenomenology, 16* (Special edition: contemporary phenomenological research on key psychotherapeutic issues), 15. doi: 10.1080/20797222.2016.1164989

Kramer, E. (2000). *Art as therapy: Collected papers.* London, England: Jessica Kingsley.

Leclerc, J. (2011). Re-presenting trauma: The witness function in the art of the Holocaust. *Art Therapy, 28*(2), 82–89. doi: 10.1080/07421656.2011.580181

Levitt, L. (2007). American Jewish loss after the Holocaust. New York, NY: New York University Press.

Makarova, E. (1990). *From Bauhaus to Terezín: Friedl Dicker-Brandeis and her pupils.* Jerusalem, Israel: Holocaust Martyrs' and Heroes' Remembrance Authority, The Art Museum.

Makarova, E. (2001). *Friedl Dicker-Brandeis.* Los Angeles, CA: Tallfellow/Ever Picture Press.

Midwest Center for Holocaust Education. (1999, September 2.) *Judy Jacobs interview.* https:// mchekc.org/wp-content/uploads/2021/01/JacobsJudyTranscript.pdf

Presiado, M. (2012). These threads captured shadows: Sewing and embroidery in Holocaust art works of contemporary Jewish women artists. *Ars Judaica, 8,* 99–118.

Presiado, M. (2015). Reconstructing life stories of Holocaust survivors through art: The case of Esther Nisenthal Krinitz and Ilana Ravek. *Journal of Modern Jewish Studies, 15*(2), 246–266.

Presiado, M. (2016). A new perspective on Holocaust art: women's artistic expression of the female Holocaust experience (1939-49), *Holocaust Studies, 22*(4), 417–446. doi: 10.1080/ 17504902.2016.1201365

Rosenberg, P. (2001). *Learning about the Holocaust through art.* http://art.holocaust-education.net/

Sartre, J-P. (1956). *Being and nothingness* (H. Barnes, trans.). New York, NY: Philosophical Library. (Original published 1943.)

Sujo, G. (2001). *Legacies of silence: The visual arts and Holocaust memory.* London, England: Philip Wilson Publishers.

Wix, L. (2003). Art in the construction of self: Three women and their ways in art, therapy and education. *Dissertation Abstracts International, 64*(02), 245. (UMI No. 3081230)

Wix, L. (2009). Aesthetic empathy in teaching art to children: The work of Friedl Dicker-Brandeis in Terezin. *Art Therapy, 26*(4), 152–158. doi: 10.1080/07421656.2009.10129612

Yad Vashem. *Interview with Yehuda Bacon, Holocaust survivor and artist.* https://www.yadvashem. org/articles/interviews/yehuda-bacon.html.

Zapruder, A. (Ed.). (2002). *Salvaged pages: Young writers' diaries of the Holocaust.* New Haven, CT: Yale University Press.

Zhavi, D. (2003). *Husserl's phenomenology.* Stanford, CA: Stanford University Press.

CHAPTER 6

NARRATIVES OF HOLOCAUST ARTISTS

I was honored to have the opportunity to meet some of the artists who had created artwork during the Holocaust. I had read about and viewed their works for years prior to commencing this study, and was eager to hear their stories directly from their voice. My intention was to conduct interviews in person, in order to immerse myself in the data (Finlay, 2009) not only by collecting verbal accounts, but also by experiencing the individual's presence. Unfortunately, time and money prohibited me from traveling to meet each individual, though I was able to conduct three semi-structured interviews in person, four via video chat and one on the phone. In each interview, I asked the participant to simply talk about their experience making art during the Holocaust. I aimed to stay within the confines of the phenomenological method, which encourages the researcher to bracket off existing information they may know about the participants or phenomenon; however, I did ask for clarification on statements they had made in the documentary or regarding artworks I was familiar with. I recorded the audio of each interview using a recording application on an iPad and took notes on participants' facial expressions, tone and other non-verbal cues when relevant.

In the following paragraphs, I elaborate on each interview and recount the extraordinary stories of each artist, based on the information obtained through interviews, as well as supplemental sources such as testimonials, texts and literature on the subject.

FREDERICK TERNA

I contacted Frederick Terna via email in August 2017 and he invited me to meet in his home in Brooklyn in early September. I spent three hours with him, learning his story and seeing his current artwork. Frederick Terna was born in Vienna, Austria, in 1923. His family moved to his father's native Prague when Terna was a child. He was forced to leave school after the Nazi occupation in 1939. He described his father as "a connected man" (F. Terna, personal communication, September 5, 2017) and was able to get forged paperwork for his family. Terna hid on a farm near Lobkovice until he was arrested by the SS in 1941 and sent to the forced labor camp Lipa. He described the SS as becoming increasingly cruel until Lipa closed in 1943. Terna was assigned transport number CV608 and, like most of the other prisoners, was sent to Terezín.

In Terezín, Terna was assigned to a unit that did maintenance work throughout the ghetto. This allowed him to walk around the ghetto more freely, a luxury he recalled abusing. He said that he was loosely connected to the artists in the design department, including professional artist Bedrich Fritta, and was able to obtain art materials from them:

> I made drawings and at one time I had the courage to go talk to Fritta and show him my things and he said, "Terrible." And I was getting smaller and smaller. He said, "It's fine work, but if they find it on you, you're dead." (F. Terna, personal communication, September 5, 2017)

DOI: 10.4324/9781003160885-9

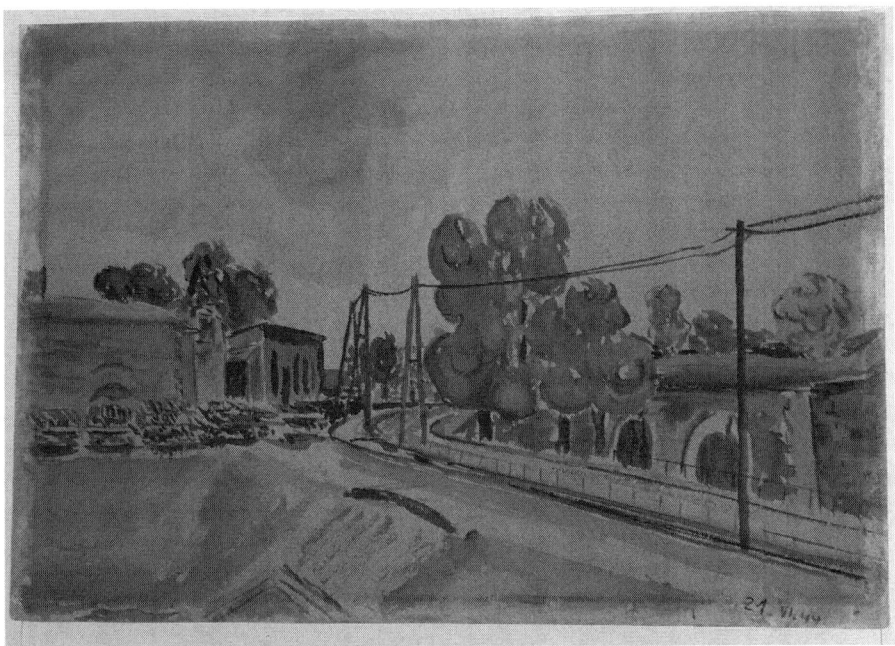

Figure 6.1 Frederick Terna (1923–). *Near the Railway.* Terezín, 1943. Courtesy of Beit Theresienstadt, Kibbutz Givat Hayim- Ihud, Israel.

Despite this warning, Terna continued to draw. He began spending time with an architect he knew, František Zelenka,[1] who showed him different techniques. He learned how to create his own ink by scraping carbon off the bottom of sinks and mixing it with water. He whittled dowels for maneuvering the ink on paper he found and kept his works hidden in a box. Terna fashioned a distinct but covert signature for himself so that, if found, the works could not be identified as his. He drew images from around the ghetto and considers this his first body of artwork: "Was it art? I don't know. It was visual information on the spot, first-hand reporting. Whether art or not is unimportant, it is visual evidence." He began to imagine himself making a career as an artist if he survived.

In 1944, Terna was sent to Auschwitz for a brief period, and then to Kaufering, a sub-camp of Dachau. The 12-hour workdays did not allow for time to draw in his barracks; nor did he have access to traditional materials. However, Terna recalled doodling with the sand he noticed while working: "Take a plank, put a bit of sand on it, take a stick, and draw in the sand. If a guard comes by, kick the sand. So there I was continuing to think about drawing. All I owned was a spoon" (F. Terna, personal communication, September 5, 2017). Because of this, Terna continues to use sand in his artwork to this day.

---

1   Of note, Zelenka designed the stage and costumes for the children's production *Brundibár,* which was performed in Terezín in September 1943.

Terna was liberated outside of Kaufering on April 27, 1945 and was eventually taken to a German displaced persons camp. He recalled a "kind soul" giving him paper and watercolors:

> I painted what I knew. Auschwitz, and other things. And then I caught myself and said, "Wait a minute, I'm out from there. I don't have to do this anymore." And I switched abruptly to landscapes. I looked out the window; by then it was spring. I painted landscapes. But it didn't take me too long to realize the landscapes had fences and walls and I realized, "It's not going to go away." And I have accepted that. This is my stance to this day: it's not going to go away. It showed then right after liberation, in my art, and it's still there to this day.

Terna made his way to Paris in 1946 and began to study art. In 1952, he moved to New York and continued to paint. In the 1980s he visited Beit Terezín. While looking through the museum archives, Terna found his own drawings from the ghetto, which he donated to Beit Terezín. On his current art process, Terna said:

> To me, painting is an unashamed service. When something bothers me, it goes in there. I am using art for selfish reasons. And it works. When I am happy, I know how to paint; when I am miserable, I know how to deal with that. And I've got all stages in between.

YEHUDA BACON

I met Yehuda Bacon in a conference room at the Leo Baeck Institute in his neighborhood in Jerusalem. He was soft spoken and kind; and as he shared his experience, I struggled to imagine this gentle man in such harsh conditions. Bacon was born in 1929 to an observant Jewish family in Ostrava, Czechoslovakia. He described the town as a melting point of three countries, where residents spoke Czech, German and Hebrew or Yiddish. In 1942, he was sent on a transport to Terezín. While waiting for the transport, known artist Leo Hass observed Bacon drawing and gave him feedback

Bacon was sent to the children's home in Terezín. In our interview, he emphasized that although there was an established children's home, not all children in the ghetto lived there: "All children were not in the children's home. Most had to sleep in the roof with the old and sick. We had it better" (Y. Bacon, personal communication, September 26, 2017). Bacon's best friend was the son of Jacob Edelstein, chairman of the ghetto's Jewish Council. This friendship allowed Bacon extra rations of bread and some degree of safety. He was also able to connect with other prominent members of the ghetto, such as the artists assigned to the design department. Otto Ungar gave Bacon short lessons on how to make images three dimensional, which he recalled feeling grateful for.

Bacon took part in unofficial art lessons with other children in the ghetto. Since education was prohibited, one child from the lesson would stand on lookout for approaching SS. The children hid their work and always had a false story prepared to tell the SS if they were caught: "If you were caught, you were destined to go on the next transport east. And you know what is east. It was a very severe punishment, no one knows what is east, just that you don't come back" (Y. Bacon, personal communication, September 26, 2017). Bacon began drawing buildings in the ghetto and was even offered a half-portion of bread as payment for a drawing. That exchange made him see himself as an artist. He continued to draw and shared his work with Dr. Karel Fleischmann, a talented artist and assistant director of the Terezín Health Department. Fleischmann told Bacon that he was a "gifted child" (Y. Bacon, personal communication, September 26, 2017). and provided him with additional art materials. Bacon learned how to draw portraits and began depicting his peers in the ghetto.

In December 1943, before the Red Cross visit to Terezín, Bacon's family was sent on a transport to Auschwitz-Birkenau. The group was kept in the family camp for six months and given special treatment in the event that the Red Cross visited the camp. Bacon recalled that the SS "wanted to have a few people more or less who looked in order. But, after their performance, they could go to the gas chambers" (Y. Bacon, personal communication, September 26, 2017). Indeed, after six months in the family camp, the majority of people on Bacon's transport were murdered in the gas chambers.

The family camp contained a specific block for children, Block 31, headed by German Jew Freddy Hirsh. Bacon credits his safety in the family camp to Hirsh, who organized education and cultural activities for the children. Bacon recalled the incongruity of these activities in Auschwitz: "You can have no education, but here is a block with children, where we can sing and dance. SS would come watch. After selection, we would do this. I lived this paradox" (Y. Bacon, personal communication, September 26, 2017). Bacon was given drawing materials, which he used to depict the world around him: "I drew my friends. And I drew a kind of hand, a cruel hand, and I thought, 'That is the hand of fate.' And I drew a *muselmann*. A lot of drawings like that—very, sick, ill people" (Y. Bacon, personal communication, September 26, 2017). Most of these drawings were lost.

In June 1944, when the family camp was liquidated, Bacon evaded death and was assigned a job with older teenage boys in the *Rollwagenkommando* (wagon command). In this role, Bacon transported items around the Auschwitz complex and was exposed to atrocities occurring throughout the camps. He witnessed transports enter and move through the selection process. In 1944, Bacon saw a fellow artist friend from Terezín, Petr Ginz, arrive on a transport:

> I saw him marching to the gas chamber. I was in Auschwitz and I knew exactly who would go to the gas chambers. I knew him, and I saw him. I couldn't speak to him, it was forbidden; but I saw him with other children marching (Y. Bacon, personal communication, September 26, 2017).

Experiences like this reminded Bacon of how precarious his existence was.

Bacon became friendly with members of the *Sonderkommando* (a taskforce of prisoners forced to work in the gas chambers) and was able to tour the gas chambers to learn how they worked. He began drawing scenes of Auschwitz, as well as portraits of people he interacted with, with the goal of commemorating their lives:

> I had a tremendous desire to remember what I saw. I knew I wouldn't get out; but you never know, "Maybe somehow I will get out, and I will tell about you." I didn't say, "I swear," but, "I promise you, with my whole heart" (Y. Bacon, personal communication, September 26, 2017).

Bacon recalled the names and numbers of his friends in the *Sonderkommando,* as their friendship had been significant to him. Though he knew drawing was dangerous, he continued to document his surroundings:

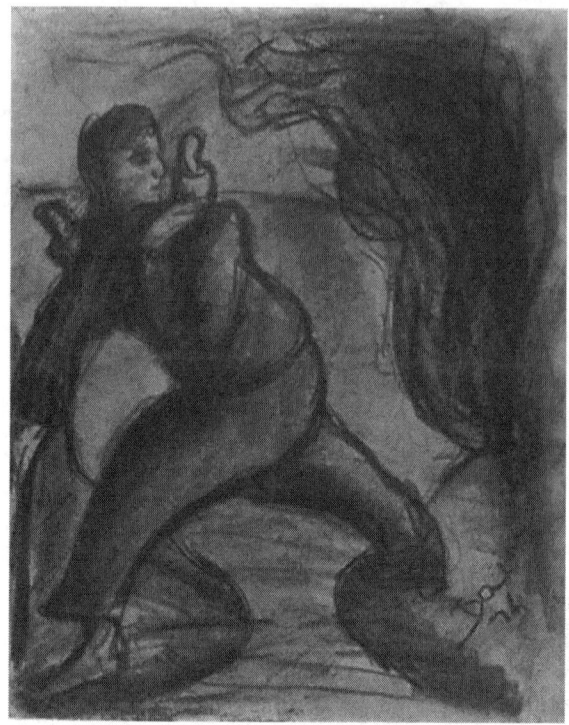

Figure 6.2 Yehuda Bacon (1929–). *Fleeing the Fire, Torah Scroll in Hand.* Auschwitz, 1945. Courtesy of the Ghetto Fighters' House Museum Art Collection, Western Galilee, Israel.

> You had to be very clever to survive. You had to be so clever and so quick. And this awareness of danger, we had to be like an animal who is hunted. If you don't see how quick the SS can come, you are gone... In Auschwitz, you never know where you will be led, who will be above you. But even in these circumstances I kept drawing. (Y. Bacon, personal communication, September 26, 2017).

After Auschwitz was liberated in 1945, Bacon returned to the gas chambers and crematoria, which he drew in impeccable detail. These drawings matched the architectural plans found in the SS technical department and were subsequently used as evidence in the Eichmann trials and the David Irving trial. Bacon also recreated many of the drawings he had made earlier in Auschwitz. With regard to his motivation for drawing after liberation, he told me:

> I wanted to be a witness. I was a child, and I thought, "What can I do? I have to be a spokesman for the children's soul which does not exist anymore." They can't tell you. I didn't know how to speak. And I could describe something in such detail that the people couldn't take it. I could tell them exactly how high the flames in the crematoria were and you can't do that—they couldn't listen; they didn't want to hear. "Well," I thought, "I could draw for myself". And from this came many, many drawings, of the shootings, crematoriums, *muselmanns*. And so on. And slowly when I started to study art, I divided it. I want to be an artist, and I said, "Well, I've done this from memory, and now I am a different person, I want to do something different." But I couldn't take away the past. (Y. Bacon, personal communication, September 26, 2017).

In an interview with Yad Vashem, Bacon explained his hope that his artwork would both educate and inspire: "For me it was a package deal: I have to tell with the intention that people will be better and such a thing will never recur" (Yad Vashem, n.d., para 31).

Like Terna, Bacon made a career as an artist. He emigrated to Israel in 1946 and studied at the Bezalel Academy of Arts and Design. He has exhibited artworks in galleries spanning the United States, Europe and Israel. He lives in Jerusalem and continues to paint.

SAMUEL BAK

I was unable to meet Samuel Bak in person, but I did interview him via Skype on October 10, 2017. Samuel Bak was born on August 12, 1933 in Vilna, Poland, to an educated, cultured Jewish family. The town fell under Soviet rule in 1939 and was then occupied by Germany in 1941. The Germans quickly established a ghetto for Jewish residents and sent Jewish males, including Bak's father, to work in a labor camp. Bak and his mother were able to hide briefly in a Benedictine convent, where a nun provided Bak with art supplies. They were caught and forced into the Vilna ghetto. The family lived in a tiny apartment and Bak's father spent most of his day at the labor site.

The creative culture was an established part of the Vilna community and that culture was maintained during German occupation. The poets Avrom Sutzkever and Szmerke Kaczerginski noticed nine-year-old Bak's interest in art and invited him to participate in an art exhibition organized by ghetto residents. Bak recalled that other artists deemed it inappropriate to include a child in the art exhibit, but he felt protected by the poets. He talked about the importance of cultural activities in the ghetto as an attempt to resist the dehumanizing conditions:

> I think it had simply to do with the fact that people were put in a situation in which they were victims of dehumanization. And within this fear in which they lived, they wanted to fight it and humanize themselves as much as possible. Out of respect for the things that they thought were important in human life, that make us more than animals—appreciation of music, appreciation of literature, of visual arts, and so on—to give it importance. And it is not perchance that it happened within the sphere of the ghetto theater. Because there, everyday something was happening. Musicians were playing jazz; can you imagine, people playing jazz in the ghetto? But they were doing it because these were the moments when people were kind of allowed to become humans (S. Bak, personal communication, October 10, 2017).

The poets also gave Bak the *Pinkus*, the official record book of the Jewish community, and encouraged him to draw in it. Bak spent the next two years filling the margins and empty pages of the *Pinkus* with his drawings. He recalled drawing images of Greek mythology, which he now views as a form of escapism: "It allowed me to go away, to go into some other world" (S. Bak, personal communication, October 10, 2017).

He also spoke about the importance of the physical book, as well as the significance of the poets gifting it to him:

> It was paper, where I could continue with my drawings, so that was very important. It was also a book that was given to me by two men who I admired. And they conveyed to me the importance of the act. When they gave the book to me, they had some

thoughts that at that age I wasn't able to grasp. That, "Maybe this child is condemned to death and he will not survive; maybe what he has to give, within the limits of what he can create, this will remain". (S. Bak, personal communication, October 10, 2017).

Bak became known as a young prodigy in the ghetto. At one point, his parents brought him clay, a material he was unfamiliar with: "It was somehow paralyzing knowing that this matter is so precious. Because in the ghetto, everything was so precious: paper, pencil. So all this brought it to a realm of importance that wouldn't have existed in a normal life" (S. Bak, personal communication, October 10, 2017).

Bak used the clay to sculpt an image of Moses. He wanted to display the sculpture in the center of the ghetto, for all residents to be reminded that the Jewish people had previously suffered persecution and were ultimately saved. "I knew that Moses was the great liberator of enslaved and oppressed Jews," Bak said, continuing, "It was he who led them out of Egypt, and therefore I figured that it would be very auspicious to create for the ghetto a sculpture in his honor" (Bak, 2001, p. 18). The sculpture did not survive, though Bak's sketches of Moses did (Figure 6.3).

The Vilna ghetto was liquidated in September 1943. Some 19,000 of the ghetto's residents were sent to death camps, while another 2,000 were kept in newly established labor camps outside of the ghetto. Bak and his parents were transported to labor camp Herren Kommando Platz, due to his father's work assignment as a welder. They lived in a cramped cell with three other people. Bak continued to draw in the

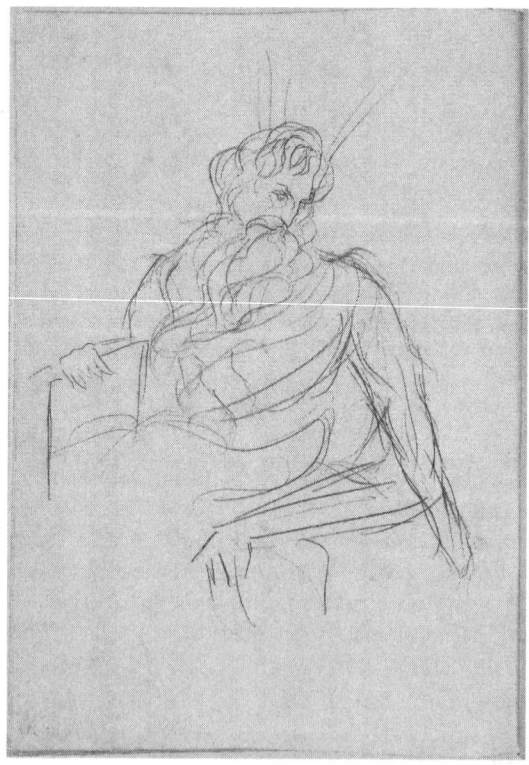

Figure 6.3 Samuel Bak (1933–). *Moses (from the Book Pinkus).* Vilna ghetto, Lithuania, 1943. Courtesy of the Vilna Gaon State Jewish Museum.

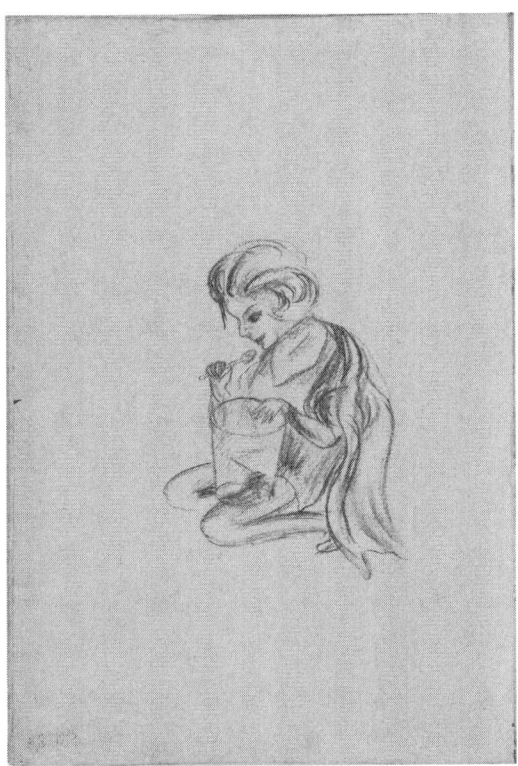

Figure 6.4 Samuel Bak (1933–). *Untitled (from the Book Pinkus)*. Vilna ghetto, Lithuania, 1943. Courtesy of the Vilna Gaon State Jewish Museum.

Pinkus, which he found to be safe and comforting. On the morning of March 27, 1944, the *Gestapo* demanded that all children be brought into the courtyard. Bak's mother hid him with two other children under a bed covered with clothing. From his hiding place, Bak heard the gunshots that killed 250 children. That night, his father quickly made arrangements for Bak and his mother to escape. His mother was snuck out of the camp immediately. Bak hid in their unit for a few days until it was confirmed that his mother had found refuge with a Catholic relative outside of the camp. His father placed him in a sack used for transporting wood and gave him directions. The sack was put on a truck leaving the camp and Bak was picked up by a woman he didn't know and brought to his mother. Bak and his mother once again hid in a convent. His father was shot with other labor prisoners in early July 1944, just before Soviet forces liberated the city.

Bak lost the *Pinkus* during his escape, but it was found by Jewish partisans after liberation. The *Pinkus* is currently housed at the Vilna Gaon State Jewish Museum, which opened a new branch in Bak's honor in November 2017. The Samuel Bak Museum holds a large collection of Bak's post-war artwork, as well as the *Pinkus*. Bak studied and worked as an artist in Germany, France and Israel before settling in Boston in 1993. He is represented by the Pucker Gallery. The Holocaust remains a theme in his artwork: "this experience is part of me, part of how I see the world" (S. Bak, personal communication, October 10, 2017).

Bak published a biography in 2001, *Painted in Words*, which he referenced through-out our interview.

JUDY JACOBS

I connected to Judy Jacobs (née Gondos) through her daughter in law, art therapist Sherri Jacobs, who works with elderly Holocaust survivors. We spoke via phone on September 1, 2017. Jacobs was born in Budapest in 1937 to a physician father and designer mother. The Zionist family lived comfortably, as Budapest was a refuge city for Slovakian, German and Austrian Jews at the beginning of the war. Zion-ist Rudolph Kasztner organized the Relief and Rescue Committee in Budapest to help Jews safely enter Hungary from neighboring countries (USHMM, 2021). In 1944, Germany occupied Hungary, enforcing new laws and restrictions on the Jew-ish community.

Kasztner began negotiating with Nazi officials, including Adolph Eichmann, offering to trade hardware and trucks for Jewish lives. While mass transports from Budapest to Auschwitz began in May 1944, Kasztner and his partners arranged for approximately 1,700 Jews to be spared. The Relief and Rescue Committee selected a cross-section of Hungarian Jews, including Jacobs and her family, to board what became known as the Kasztner train. The train left Budapest on June 30, 1944 and was supposed to take passengers to safety in Switzerland, but was rerouted by Eich-mann to the Bergen-Belsen camp. On July 8, at age seven, Jacobs was registered in the Hungarian camp at Bergen-Belsen, where she was interned with other passengers for six months.

Jacobs recalled that their transport was treated slightly better than other prisoners:

> We were fed 350 calories per day. We didn't have to work; they didn't take away our belongings; we were allowed to mingle. We weren't physically abused, but verbally, very much so. There was a good-sized group of doctors in the camp that could use their brain power (J. Jacobs, personal communication, September 1, 2017).

Initially Jacobs and her family felt optimistic; but as days passed and the weather worsened, morale declined.

Noticing the dark mood, Jacob's mother organized spontaneous art lessons for the children in their barracks:

> One morning after roll call, my mother let out the word that any child who wanted an art class could come to our barracks. The weather wasn't too cold. Everyone was told to get a stick and draw in the dirt at their feet. They drew butterflies and flowers, none of which were things we would ever see at Bergen-Belsen. After 30 minutes or so, all the kids had drawn something and they gladly showed their masterpieces. They left happy and smiling and agreed to have class again the next day. The mood was low, dark, very depressed. It was unusual to be happy and smiling (J. Jacobs, personal communication, September 1, 2017).

The art lessons occurred a few times over the family's internment. Jacobs did not think the endeavor was particularly risky, since their group was given a degree of preferential treatment. She recalled the experience being more significant for her mother:

My mother decided to do the class because it was something that she knew how to do. Everyone was very despondent, and she felt that if she could distract them and lift their morale, then she would have accomplished something. And it worked. The kids had their morale boosted and so did my mother. She had done something positive (J. Jacobs, personal communication, September 1, 2017).

I asked if she thought the classes gave her mother a sense of meaning, to which Jacobs emphatically replied: "Absolutely. It absolutely gave her a sense of meaning. And a sense of purpose" (J. Jacobs, personal communication, September 1, 2017)

Jacobs remembered another artist on their transport, Istvan Irsai, who also drew in the camp:

He was sick and my father was a doctor, so he saw him. And he realized that this artist was okay, just starving. So my father arranged for him to get an extra ration of bread. And he drew a little picture for him of a piece of bread with a thermometer in it, since that had been the prescription. He used small pieces of cardboard. I guess he did that for two reasons. One, he liked making art. Two, maybe he felt like he needed to compensate those who did for him (J. Jacobs, personal communication, September 1, 2017).

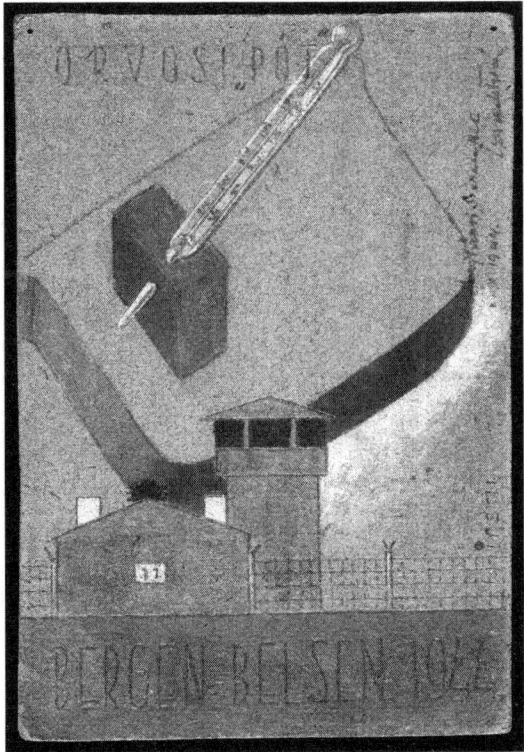

Figure 6.5 Istvan Irsai (1896–1968). *Bergen-Belsen 1944 (A Gift to Dr. Gondos).* Bergen-Belsen, 1944. United States Holocaust Memorial Museum, courtesy of Bela Gondos.

After a six-month internment, the passengers of the Kasztner transport boarded a train to freedom. Their transport was taken out of Bergen-Belsen in December 1944 and arrived in Switzerland on Christmas Eve. The refugees were treated by the Swiss and International Red Cross at a hotel in Montreux. Jacob's mother continued to teach art to the refugee children while her father tried to figure out how to practice medicine again. The family spent a few months in Geneva before immigrating to the United States in 1946. They lived between Washington DC and Boston. Jacobs attended college, where she met her husband, and eventually settled in Kansas City.

HALINA OLOMUCKI

Early in my inquiry, I came across the artwork of Polish artist Halina Olomucki. Olomucki survived the war, but passed away in 2007 at age 88. I was disappointed that I had missed the opportunity to speak directly with her, but was able to connect with her daughter, Miriam Alon. Although not a survivor herself, Alon has written and given presentations about her mother, and has boxes of Olomucki's artworks and writings. Alon and I communicated via email before meeting at her home in Ashkelon, Israel, for a formal interview about her mother's experience.

Halina Olomucki was born to a Jewish family in Warsaw, Poland in 1919. She showed an interest in art at a young age. In 1939, after the German occupation of Poland, her family was moved to the Warsaw ghetto, where Olomucki continued to draw whenever possible: "Of course there were no paints and colors, but always a pencil and always a piece of paper somewhere. My main job was to observe, I was always good at observation" (as cited in Rosenberg, 2001). Olomucki worked outside of the ghetto and was able to give her drawings to a man she met who kept them safe.

In May 1943, Olomucki and her family were detained in the *Umschlagplatz*, an area outside of the ghetto that was designated to hold people before transport to the death camps. That was the last place Olomucki saw her family. She was transported to the Majdanek camp, certain she would die. At one point, the head of her block asked if anyone knew how to paint. Olomucki volunteered and was soon commissioned to create signs around the barracks for the Germans. In return, Olomucki was offered extra rations of bread. She saved the art materials she was given and began creating her own artwork, which she hid. The artwork consisted mostly of portraits and scenes of the women around her.

Later in 1943, Olomucki was sent to Auschwitz-Birkenau. She worked in a union command with other young women and was again asked to create signs and other works for her captors. She continued to make her own clandestine art. The women around her requested that she draw them: "'If you live to leave this hell, make your drawings and tell the world about us. We want to remain among the living, at least on paper" (as quoted in Novitch, Dawidowicz & Freudenheim, 1981, p. 17). Alon elaborated on this quote, stating: "They said that she has to survive, to paint them, so that people won't forget them" (M. Alon, personal communication, September 25, 2017). In an oral testimony, Olomucki described her need to draw:

> My observation, my need to observe what was going on, was stronger than my body. It was a need, a driving need. It was the most important. I never thought rationally what I am doing, but I had this incredible need to draw, to write down what was happening. I was in the same condition as every other person all around me, I saw them close to death but I never thought of myself close to death. I was in the air. I was outside my existence. My job was simply to write down, to draw what was happening (as cited in Rosenberg, 2001, para 7).

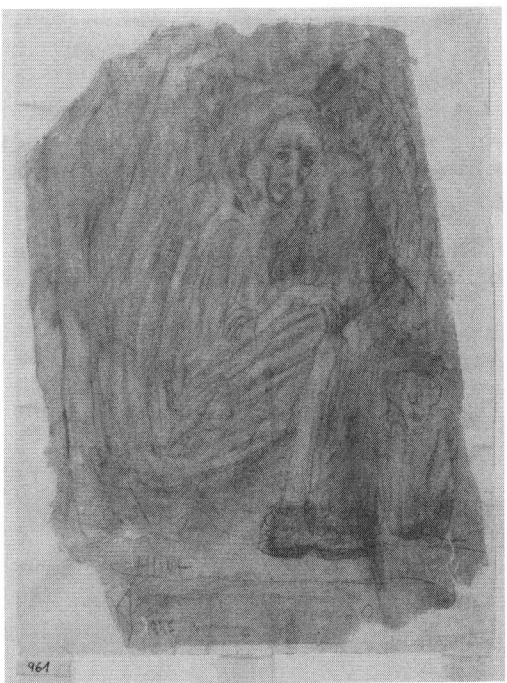

Figure 6.6 Halina Olomucki (1919–2007). *Women in the Birkenau Camp.* Auschwitz-Birkenau, 1945. Courtesy of the Ghetto Fighters' House Museum Art Collection, Western Galilee, Israel.

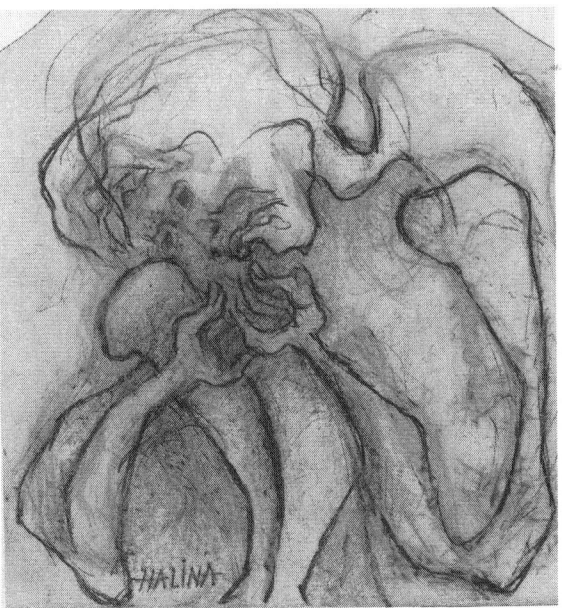

Figure 6.7 Halina Olomucki (1919–2007). *The Hunger.* Auschwitz-Birkenau, 1943–1945. Courtesy of the United States Holocaust Memorial Museum.

Alon reflected on her mother's need to create, despite the inherent risks: "When they give her a way to draw or paint something for them, it was also a way to do so for herself" (M. Alon, personal communication, September 25, 2017). She continued: "But the moment they caught her, it was death on the spot. But for her, it wasn't like playing with fire. If she didn't do that, she had no purpose. It was exactly like breathing." Olomucki was known as an artist and her daughter believes that the artistic identity saved her spirit:

> I think it was her identity… It was such a big part of her that without that, she would have to find another way. But it was such a big part of her identity that I think—I am almost sure—that if she didn't draw, she would lose herself (M. Alon, personal communication, September 25, 2017).

Olomucki was evacuated on a death march beginning on January 18, 1945. She spent a brief period in Ravensbrück and was then transferred to the sub-camp Neustadt-Glewe, where she was liberated on May 2, 1945. She continued to draw during the liberation period and later returned to Birkenau to recover her hidden works. She moved back to Warsaw and married another Holocaust survivor, architect Boleslan Olomucki. The couple moved to Lodz, where Olomucki took classes at the Fine Arts Academy. She studied under the avant-garde painter Władysław Strzemiński, then moved to Paris in 1957. In 1972, Olomucki, her husband and daughter Miriam settled in Israel, where she lived until her death from Alzheimer's in 2007.

HELGA HOŠKOVÁ-WEISSOVÁ

I had come across the name Helga Hošková while reading about Holocaust artwork, but had not sought her out. I had made the incorrect assumption that since she was a young female adolescent in Terezín, she had worked under Friedl Dicker-Brandeis. Because the aim of my study was artists who created on their own accord, and because Friedl's name was already known in art therapy literature, I did not initially pursue a meeting with Hošková-Weissová. However, when a curator from Beit Terezín offered to put me in touch with her, I did not waste the opportunity.

I interviewed Hošková-Weissová via Skype on January 22, 2021. She was emphatic that although she lived in L-410, the girls' home where Friedl taught, she had not been involved in her classes: "She (Friedl) wanted to keep children away from the terrible situations, but with my drawings I wanted to say something" (H. Hošková-Weissová, personal communication, January 22, 2021). Hošková-Weissová was motivated to draw by her father, who had encouraged her to draw the scenes around her in the ghetto. Throughout our interview, she held images of her artwork up to the screen to provide further details and explanations of her experience. I later purchased her published diary, which contains many of the images she created in captivity, to supplement our interview.

Helga Hošková-Weissová was born to a Jewish family in Prague on November 10, 1929. She was dismissed from fourth grade after the German occupation and began keeping a diary of her experiences under Nazi rule as they unfolded. She described the fear she and her friends felt as former classmates were sent on transports, up until she and her family received their own notice. The family was sent to Terezín on December 7, 1941. Each individual was allowed to bring 50 kilograms of luggage.

Hošková-Weissová made sure to pack her watercolors, crayons and sketchbook, along with her diary.

In Terezín, Hošková-Weissová and her mother were assigned to a women's barracks while her father was assigned to a men's workforce. She sent her father a drawing of two children building a snowman, to which he replied: "Draw what you see." In response, Hošková-Weissová made over 100 drawings and paintings depicting daily life during her three years in Terezín. She documented the harsh realities of the ghetto in drawings of crowded barracks and lines for food. She expressed the daily fear of being sent on a transport east in a drawing of a ghetto leader bringing a transport notice at night. But in addition, Hošková-Weissová documented the cultural community that thrived with the ghetto, with drawings depicting concerts, lessons and Jewish rituals. She said that drawing allowed her to escape into her own world where no one could enter.

Hošková-Weissová shared that her father wrote a poem and dedicated it to the leader of the Czech Philharmonic orchestra, who was also captive in the Terezín ghetto. The poem included the line: "play to us, and make us well again, we must live each moment to the full. If we don't, die like cattle." His words illustrate the need for cultural activity to help ghetto residents retain a sense of humanity in order to persevere. Like her father, Hošková-Weissová clung to her own identity through her drawing and journaling.

Hošková-Weissová and her mother were put on a transport to Auschwitz in October 1944. Before they left, Hošková-Weissová gave her drawings to her uncle, who hid them in a brick wall in the ghetto. Upon arrival in Auschwitz, she was able to pass as older than 15 and was therefore considered eligible for work. After just ten days, the mother and daughter were sent to a subcamp of the Flossenbürg labor camp, where they worked in an aircraft factory: "We were all seeded for murder, but they [the Germans] used our strength." Hošková-Weissová and her mother were evacuated to Mauthausen in April 1945, a journey that took 16 days. They were liberated there on May 5, 1945. The pair returned to Prague later that month and were able to move back into their apartment. Her father never returned.

Hošková-Weissová attended high school and studied art in Prague. In 1958, she illustrated Holocaust survivor Arnošt Lustig's first book, *Night and Hope*. In the 1960s, she began a series titled *Calvary*, inspired by her experiences in Terezín, Auschwitz and Flossenbürg. The paintings were exhibited across Prague, Italy and Germany. She studied art briefly in Israel before returning to Prague, where she still lives.

THOMAS GEVE

A curator at the Yad Vashem art museum emailed me a link to Thomas Geve's website and recommended I reach out to him for an interview. I sent an email through the website in late 2020 and was answered by Geve's daughter, Yifat Cohn-Meir. Yifat, who lives in Israel, was in the process of republishing her father's testimony and drawings, and was available via Zoom for multiple interviews. Though she lives close to her father's assisted living community, the COVID-19 pandemic limited their ability to meet in person, and she worried that he might not be able to schedule and execute a Zoom meeting without her assistance. Therefore, I compiled a list of questions for Geve, which she asked him over the phone and then reported the answers back to me in our conversations. Luckily, Geve called Yifat during one of our interviews and I had the opportunity to speak directly to him as well.

Thomas Geve was born in 1929 in Szczecin, Germany, now part of Poland. When Hitler came to power in 1933, Geve's father, a surgeon, lost his practice and the family moved to his father's home town of Beuthen. Beuthen was a mining town on the border of Poland and Germany where both Polish and German were spoken. As antisemitism increased, Geve's father began making plans for his family to emigrate to England. In the summer of 1939, Geve's father left for England to establish himself before sending for his wife and son. Geve moved to Berlin in the interim. Geve enjoyed sketching the buildings he saw in Berlin, though he did not consider himself an artist. In his 1958 autobiography, *Youth in Chains*, republished in 1987 as *Guns and Barbed Wire: A Child Survives the Holocaust*, Geve recalled the food ration cards that German Jews were forced to use, as well as the yellow stars they were forced to wear.

In late June 1943, Geve and his mother were sent on a transport to Auschwitz-Birkenau. The two were separated upon arrival. Geve, not yet 14 years old, was placed in quarantine and eventually put in a men's camp, Auschwitz I, in the bricklaying school barracks. He was one of the youngest boys in the bricklaying unit, a job that he believes saved his life. Geve saw his mother once in the camp—a brief encounter that he says "kept me going." He decided he needed to plan an escape and began sketching clandestinely. When possible, he peeled off the layers of paper that the cement at his worksite was wrapped in and saved them for drawings. He sketched the environment around him and made lists of the guards and their duty stations to strategize his escape. Geve drew maps of the camp complex and surrounding areas, though he ultimately did not execute his plan. Making these sketches gave him a sense of control which was otherwise impossible in the camp. When we spoke, he explained that "being and doing is a very strong thing for the spirit." Geve hid his sketches and lists in sacks of straw, but they were lost when Auschwitz was evacuated.

Geve's mother was killed in Auschwitz-Birkenau. In January 1945, Geve survived a 60-kilometer death march and was then transported briefly to Gross-Rosen, followed by Buchenwald. He was unable to procure sketching materials in Buchenwald; nor did he have a place to hide drawings if he did access any. He spent two and a half months completing grueling manual labor until the camp was liberated on April 11, 1945.

As a teenager with nowhere to go, Geve stayed in Buchenwald with the Allied forces, who brought food and medication. Former prisoners organized the remaining inmates into blocks according to language and nationality, and Geve was placed in a German-speaking block along with the historian Eugen Kogon. The American liberation forces asked the survivors to collect Nazi paperwork and other documents from around Buchenwald. Geve was too weak to walk around the camp, so he stayed back and began drawing what he remembered as his own form of documentation. In our interview, his daughter explained that some survivors didn't know how to write or lacked the mental capacity to put into words what they had experienced, so drawing was an appropriate alternative. In his autobiography, Geve elaborated: "We did not want to forget. On the contrary, we felt an urge to set what we had witnessed on paper and to tell about it. I, too, was gripped by that desire" (1987, p. 205). He continued: "If we who had experienced it, I reasoned, did not expose the bitter truth, people simply would not believe about the Nazi ogre." Using abandoned Nazi postcards and bits of colored pencils, Geve detailed his imprisonment, from entering Auschwitz's

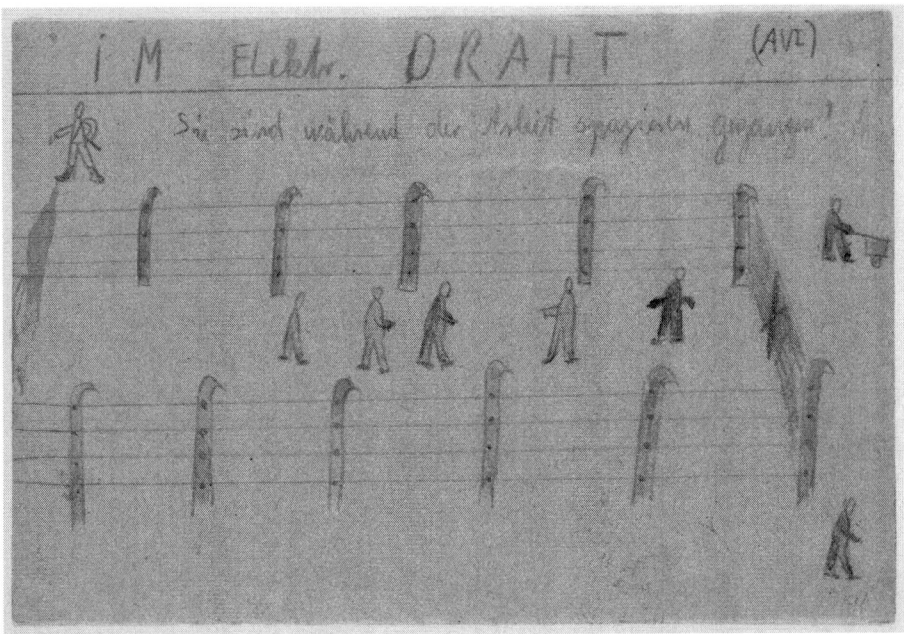

Figure 6.8 Thomas Geve (1929–). *Between the Electrified Wires*. Buchenwald displaced persons camp, 1945. Pencil, colored pencil and watercolor on paper, 10 × 15 cm. Collection of the Yad Vashem Art Museum, Jerusalem. Gift of the artist. Photo © Yad Vashem Art Museum, Jerusalem.

quarantine to liberation. He wrote that these scenes "became vivid again – the arrival, the selection, the punishments, the food, the diseases, the endless rows of fencing, the work, the roll calls, the winter, the revolts, the gallows, the evacuation, the Katushas" (1987, p. 205). An American soldier noticed Geve's drawings and gave him a pack of watercolors, which Geve used to bring more color to what he described as a "colorless place." He felt a sense of pride that the color in his artwork provided more detailed evidence than the black and white photographs that the Allied forces took (Figure 6.8).

In his most recent autobiography, *The Boy Who Drew Auschwitz* (2021), Geve expounded on the impulse to draw in the days preceding liberation:

> The experience of 22 months of my life in three concentration camps was just waiting to burst out from my restless brain. Depicting the dark, sad, colourless life in the camps in all the seven colours of the rainbow made my heart rejoice and spurred me on. Those creations, in honour and memory of my friends and comrades, became another precious victory (p. 280)

Geve was motivated to find his father and show him his drawings to share what he had endured. In June 1945, the International Red Cross sent 107 adolescent boys from Buchenwald, including Geve, to the Felsenegg children's home on the Zugerberg mountain, overlooking Zug, Switzerland. A teacher noticed Geve drawing his experiences from the camps, as well as the sense of purpose he attained from drawing, and encouraged the other boys to do the same. Drawing became quite common and the home's staff preserved the boys' artwork, knowing that it was important testimony. In 2018, the Zug Museum exhibited 150 drawings of the "Buchenwald Boys" created in the Felsenegg home detailing their war experiences.

Geve was able to locate his father in August 1945. He stayed with a Swiss family while arrangements were made for him to go to England. Geve reunited with his father in November 1945 and shared his 80-plus drawings depicting his experience. In a June 2021 Zoom lecture, Geve said: "I was excited to show my father, a surgeon, my drawings. He studied the inside of human beings and I studied the outside." His father kept the drawings in a safe and years later, Geve donated them to Yad Vashem.

Geve attended school and studied to be an engineer. In 1950, he moved to Israel and served in the Israeli Defense Force before beginning a career in engineering. He married and had three children. Geve gives frequent lectures about his Holocaust experience and the artwork he created in response. He talks about taking his "little blue friends" with him, referring to the blue he used to color in the prisoner uniforms as representations of his comrades who perished. Though the original drawings are small, Geve enjoys seeing them enlarged via projector when speaking; he feels as though he is bringing them back to life. His daughter shared that he becomes emotional "seeing his friends in full size."

ALICE EHRMANN SHEK

While conducting interviews in Israel in September 2017, I made a point to visit Beit Terezín, per Frederick Terna's suggestion. Established in 1975 on Kibbutz Givat Haim Ihud, Beit Terezín is a museum and educational center honoring the Jewish martyrs of the Terezín ghetto. I had the pleasure of seeing artwork made by artists I had previously read about, such as Leo Haas, Otto Ungar, Bedrich Fritta and Jo Spier. A curator suggested I also look at the artwork of Alice Ehrmann Shek, an artist prominently featured in the Beit Terezín archives. At the time I was unable to include Ehrmann Shek in my study, but I reached out to Beit Terezín again in early 2021. I was put in touch with Ehrmann Shek's daughter and niece, Rachel Shek and Ruthie Ofek respectively, who live in Israel.

I interviewed Shek and Ofek on January 29, 2021, via Zoom. They were able to share information on Alice Ehrmann Shek's experience in Terezín and kindly sent me a German and Hebrew copy of Ehrmann Shek's published diary. They also introduced me to Holocaust scholar Alexandra Zapruder, who translated sections of Alice's diary and other Holocaust diaries for her book, *Salvaged Pages*. Through these sources, as well as testimony courtesy of Beit Terezín, I was able to construct an understanding of Alice's experience creating artwork in Terezín.

Alice Ehrmann was born in Prague in 1927 to a Jewish father and Christian mother. Neither she nor her older sister Ruth was given a Jewish education, as the family lived a secular life. Both parents were artistic and Alice demonstrated artistic ability as a child. When the Nazis occupied Prague in 1938, they enforced the Nuremberg Race Laws, which classified Alice and Ruth as *Mischlinge* of the first degree, meaning they were half-Jewish (Zapruder, 2015). Because they were half-Jewish, the sisters quickly lost their privileges as Czech citizens. Alice was forced to leave school and in 1942 became involved in an underground Zionist youth movement, where she first met Ze'ev Shek. On July 13, 1943, she and her sister were sent to Terezín without their parents. In 1944, her father was arrested in Prague and sent to Terezín's Small Fortress, and later to Auschwitz. Her mother remained in Prague throughout the war.

Alice began drawing the scenes around her. According to her daughter, she used drawing as a form of escape: "It was her dreamland, a place where she was happy" (R. Shek, personal communication, January 29, 2021). Like other Holocaust artists, Alice drew secretly, but she also preferred to be away from even her fellow ghetto residents when doing so: "She was able to get herself into an attic to be completely alone while she drew." Alice sketched the people around her, as well as the barracks.

Alice was assigned a job as a goose herd. She reconnected with Ze'ev Shek, who was also imprisoned in Terezín. They formed a romantic relationship, which was interrupted in October 1944 when Ze'ev was sent on a transport to Auschwitz. Ze'ev had been collecting documents of the Germans' treatment of ghetto residents, which he saved in a suitcase. Prior to his transport to Auschwitz, he tasked Alice with continuing this work to ensure there was detailed evidence of the Nazis' crimes. She collected paperwork daily, which she hid in the same suitcase. Alice also began writing a diary, "to bear witness as best I can so that it will survive me" (as cited in Zapruder, 2015, p. 396). Alice wrote her diary entries in German, but used Hebrew letters to further conceal her words. She illustrated her diary entries too, and often hid other drawings in the pages.

Of the 150,000 Jews who were sent to Terezín, Alice was one of the few who remained there for the duration of the war. Some 17,000 individuals were liberated by the Red Cross in May 1945, including prisoners sent to Terezín from death camps in the weeks prior to liberation. Alice's artworks and diary therefore offer a unique perspective of the final year of the Terezín ghetto. At age 17, she wrote poignantly about the despair and exhaustion of ghetto life: "We live holding our breaths. We don't wait – we endure. I live as if at the brink of finality" (as cited in Zapruder, 2002, p. 406). She also recounted the hopelessness she felt: "it is so hard to find the strength to live one's life to the end, without simply letting oneself be killed…" (as cited in Zapruder, 2015, p. 407). She documented her thoughts in witnessing the transports of death camp survivors being brought to Terezín as the Allied forces approached and camps were liquidated: "Women, too, arrived by foot this afternoon. Eight days under way. All crippled, shrunken beings with tiny heads and burning eyes. Hunger, animal fear, insanity. In striped uniforms, barefoot…" (as cited in Zapruder, 2002, p. 415.) She also wrote about the Nazis' destruction of the evidence of their crimes, including administrative documents and files: "I watched as thousands of documents flew up in flames… I saw the numbers, digits, dates, and names of which our misery is composed, in which it is mirrored, flicker dully and turn to ashes. Who can comprehend this?" (as cited in Zapruder, 2002, p. 399). Alice's drawings, like her writing, bear witness to a broad ghetto experience that most did not live to see.

Alice and Ruth left Terezín in June 1945 and reunited with their mother in Prague. Their father had also survived and returned to the family soon after. Ruth, who had worked with typhus patients in Terezín, became ill with polio and died in

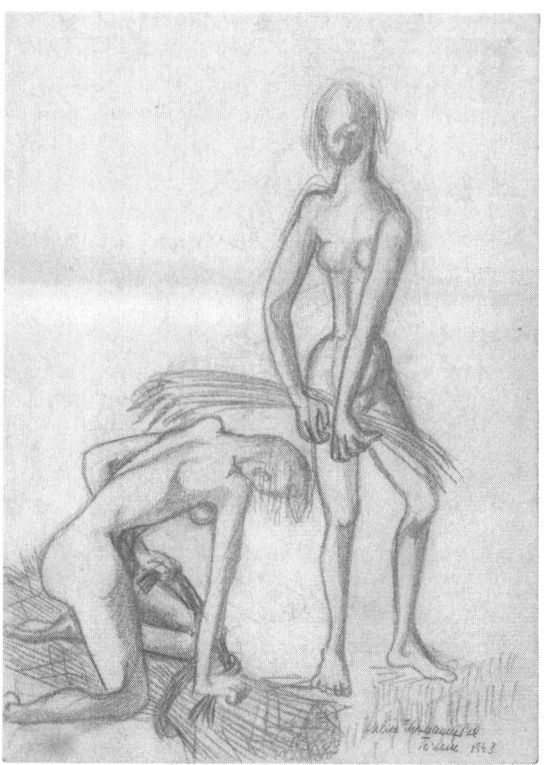

Figure 6.9 Alice Ehrmann Shek (1927–2007). *Untitled.* Terezín, 1943. Courtesy of the artist's family.

Prague later that year. Alice received news that Ze'ev had perished, which led her to despair. However, she checked the daily list of survivors posted by the Prague Jewish community until she found his name. Ze'ev was rescued by American soldiers in Dachau and returned to Prague to find Alice. The two married in 1947 and emigrated to Israel a year later. Alice worked as a set designer and illustrator, and continued to make art until her death in 2007. The couple were also among the founders of Beit Terezín, where Alice's original diary and much of her artwork are archived.

Rachel and Ruthi recalled Alice's commitment to art, noting that "it held her together" (R. Shek, personal communication, January 29, 2021). Rachel spoke about the abundance of artwork Alice created in 1946 in response to her experience. They view drawing as Alice's haven, from her time in Terezín to her death.

CONCLUSIONS

In closing this chapter, I would like to reiterate how grateful I am to the artists and their kin who took the time to speak with me in such depth. I feel fortunate to have met with or spoken to them, as our conversations were invaluable. This research would not have been possible without their participation, and I greatly appreciate their willingness to share their stories and their artworks with me.

REFERENCES

Bak, S. (2001). *Painted in words.* Bloomington, IN: Indiana University Press.

Finlay, L. (2011). *Phenomenology for therapists: Researching the lived world.* Hoboken, NJ: John Wiley and Sons.

Geve, T., Inglefield, C. (2021). *The boy who drew Auschwitz: a powerful true story of hope and survival.* London, England: Harper.

Geve, T. (1987). *Guns and barbed wire: A child Survives the Holocaust (2ndeds).* Chicago, IL: Academy Chicago Publishers.

Novitch, M., Dawidowicz, L. S. & Freudenheim, T. L. (1981). *Spiritual resistance: Art from concentration camps, 1940–1945: A selection of drawings and paintings from the collection of Kibbutz Lohamei Haghetaot, Israel.* Philadelphia, PA: Jewish Publication Society.

Rosenberg, P. (2001). *Learning about the Holocaust through art.* http://art.holocaust-education.net/

Zapruder, A. (ed.). (2002). *Salvaged pages: Young writers' diaries of the Holocaust.* New Haven, CT: Yale University Press.

CHAPTER 7

THE PHENOMENOLOGICAL INQUIRY AND RESULTS

After conducting interviews with Holocaust artists and their kin, I was left with hours of narrative transcripts to address. Prior to collecting my data, I had decided to use Amedeo Giorgi's descriptive phenomenological psychological method (2009) of analysis. Derived from Husserl's phenomenological philosophy, this method is used to describe, rather than interpret, a phenomenon. The emphasis in this methodology is on how an individual experienced the phenomenon and their subjective perspective of it (Giorgi, 2009). According to Giorgi (2012), the phenomenological inquiry "wants to understand how phenomena present themselves to consciousness and the elucidation of this process is a descriptive task" (p. 4). That is, in order to fully comprehend how individuals experience a phenomenon, the researcher must collect narrative information from those involved in the phenomenon of interest. The researcher analyzes their data using a specific protocol in order to write a description of the phenomenon. The description of the phenomenon is the summation of the researcher's results.

The descriptive phenomenological psychological method leads the researcher through five specific steps. I followed these steps as closely as possible, though I took some liberties as needed. The first step requires that the researcher assume the phenomenological attitude, which is done by bracketing off any pre-existing knowledge or expectations. Giorgi (2009, 2012) is adamant that the researcher must not bring any information apart from present data into the analysis. I attempted to assume the phenomenological attitude during my data collection, though I could not fully commit to it. My first challenge with adopting this attitude came from my insecurities as a researcher, which is a difficulty I imagine most novice researchers must contend with. I had set high expectations, both for myself and for the study, given that I was conducting it for my dissertation. I was also enthused about this research and the opportunities to interview these artists. I had expectations that participants would provide a wealth of information on their experience of making art within the Holocaust—especially since, in some cases, I had traveled across the globe to conduct interviews with them. I was eager for my interviews to satisfy my curiosity on the subject and elucidate insight into the phenomenon that I was so passionate about.

The more challenging aspect of assuming the phenomenological attitude was bracketing off my pre-existing knowledge of the phenomenon, since I was already immersed in the subject. Prior to beginning this study, I had seen many of these artworks in live exhibitions—an experience that was both inspiring and haunting. As a viewer, I paid attention to the nuances of the artworks, such as paper quality and size; the intensity of pencil marks and brush strokes; and the markings that came through the reverse side of the image. I imagined a camp prisoner leaning over a tiny scrap of paper, trying to express the enormity of their situation on such a small, flimsy surface. I thought about how the scrounged materials—ones that would be discarded in most studios—were the only tools of expression and autonomy these prisoners had. I was awestruck by the energy that was put into these works when the artists themselves were weak and starving.

DOI: 10.4324/9781003160885-10

It was impossible to fully bracket off my knowledge and perceptions of the artwork that I had seen and read about. Instead, I focused my attention on the conversations I had engaged in with the participating artists. After completing the interviews, I listened to my recordings and transcribed each one by hand in order to relive the interviews and note subtleties such as changes in tone, intakes of breath or long pauses. I set my assumptions aside and, in the second step of the method, allowed myself to read the transcripts with a clear and open mind, free of any assumptions or agendas.

The third step of Giorgi's method is to identify meaning units in order to condense the data into what is directly relevant. Giorgi (2009, 2012) advises the researcher to mark each point in the transcripts in which they experience a shift in meaning. This step became challenging, as each of my participants periodically spoke tangentially during our interviews. I noticed many shifts in my transcripts, such as when a participant detailed a specific person or place. In a supportive fashion, each participant suggested literature to read or additional artists for me to research. Some of the participants also frequently alternated between the experience of making art during and after the Holocaust. To annotate each shift would not have been efficient.

I modified the method by rereading my transcripts and noting language, recurring themes and other underlying characteristics that stood out. Though I was fascinated by each participant's account, I ignored their description of anything outside of art making in order to remain attuned to the specific phenomenon. I noted when the tone shifted from angry to nostalgic, from helpless to empowered. I also highlighted seemingly odd word choices. For example, when discussing his transport from the Terezín ghetto to Auschwitz, Yehuda Bacon said he brought his artwork along, but "it perished" (Y. Bacon, personal communication, September 26, 2017). His use of the word *perished* stood out; in the context of the Holocaust, *perished* is typically reserved for people, not items. It occurred to me that in describing his artwork as *perishing*, Bacon indicated the tremendous importance he placed on it, suggesting that he equated it with a living being. I continued this process of "lingering and amplifying" (Finlay, 1999, p. 303) on language and tone, which forced me to once again slow down and indulge in the nuances of my interviews.

The fourth step of Giorgi's method is to transform the meaning units into psychologically sensitive descriptive expressions. Giorgi (2009) recommended that the researcher use a third-person perspective to reinforce that they are analyzing someone else's experience and not their own. Since I wanted to understand the essence of the act of art making, I decided to assume the perspective of the actual artwork, as if it were hanging on the wall overseeing each interview. I did not visualize a specific piece of art, which might have taken me away from the interview and brought in pre-existing knowledge; instead, I imagined what a work by the artist could potentially hold. Reflecting on the meaning units I had identified, I considered how the artwork would respond to our conversation. Would it, for example, say, "Yes, I did represent those you lost," or "I was the only source of comfort you had"? I wrote out one to two brief descriptive statements from the perspective of the artwork for each interview, and then reduced each description into a concise existential-phenomenological statement (Table 7.1).

Once these statements were identified, I tested their internal validity through imaginative variation (Giorgi, 2009; Giorgi & Giorgi, 2003; Kapitan, 2018). I wrote and rewrote each statement multiple times, on each occasion varying the frame of reference and wording while also considering whether they were applicable to more than one participant. I noted whenever a variation altered the meaning, or essence,

Table 7.1 Existential-phenomenological statements

You need me to define yourself as human.
I am all you know and am your only constant in this landscape of uncertainty.
I am a reminder of your experiences and I will always be with you.
I affirmed your existence.
I gave you light.
I gave you a purpose
I keep you safe
I connect you to others

of the statement. Giorgi (2009) noted that the meaning "collapses" when words that describe it are not aligned with its essence. The subtleties in word choice allowed me to pinpoint precise meanings.

The fifth and final step in the data analysis is to synthesize the general psychological structure of the phenomenon (Giorgi, 2009; Kapitan, 2018). The psychological structure does not objectively define the phenomenon, but instead depicts how the phenomenon was lived based on the participants' subjective accounts (Giorgi, 2009, 2012). In describing the phenomenon, the psychological structure answers the phenomenological research question and therefore provides the results of the study. Although the psychological structure is developed through individual accounts, it is assumed to be thematically generalizable—that is, as applicable, in theory, to multiple individuals involved in the phenomenon.

RESULTS

The purpose of this study was to understand the experience of creating art during the Holocaust for a sample of survivors and second-generation survivors. Table 7.2 presents the results, beginning with the nine descriptive third-person statements; the variables that were identified in the interpretive process of imaginal variation; and their synthesis into a general psychological structure of the phenomenon. The following summary statement describes the experience of creating artwork in camps and ghettos during the Holocaust:

> Creating artwork in a camp or ghetto became a responsibility to serve as a witness because the artwork might become the only remaining witness. The physical act of art making, and the resulting work, proved that the artist existed, even if no one else did. The artwork promised a legacy in the midst of annihilation. In a landscape of uncertainty, with a constant threat of death, the art-making process became a constant, standing in for lost relationships and cementing the bonds of those relationships. Despite the great risk if caught, art making allowed artists to transcend danger and experience a degree of safety in doing something familiar and comfortable. The act of creating gave the artists a sense of beauty and served as a reminder that beauty and brightness could exist in the world. The artist identity was critical in distinguishing the artists from other captives; it nourished their spirit and allowed them to stay human. It gave them a newfound sense of purpose. The artwork that remains, even if only in the artists' memories, is a reminder of what they endured and is proof of their humanness in the face of such cruelty.

Table 7.2 Results of the phenomenological data analysis of the Holocaust artists

Existential-phenomenological statement from the perspective of the artwork	Imaginative variation	Summary statement of essence
I am burdened with the tremendous responsibility of witnessing what happened.	• I have a duty to serve as a witness. • I have a responsibility to share what I saw. • I am motivated by a desire to be a witness. • I must live, so that I can be a witness for those who didn't. • If I am not a witness, who will be? • I exist, and others do not, so I am the only witness. • I am heavy with these memories.	The artist and artwork were both physically frail and small, but carried the responsibility to be a witness. Both existed to serve as a witness.
You need me to define yourself as human.	• You rely on me. • You require me. • I help you become human. • I give you a sense of humanity. • I take away your humanity. • You want me to make you human. • I distinguish you as human. • I give you an opportunity to feel like a human again. • Without me, you are just a shell.	Being an artist distinguished an individual from others. Art making was an identity and a need beyond the basic needs for survival, making the artist a more complex, dynamic being.
I am all you know and am your only constant in this landscape of uncertainty.	• I am familiar when nothing else is. • You don't know what to expect, but you know how to make me. • You exist when I exist. • You know me, but nothing else. • I make everything more familiar.	There is a comfort in doing something familiar, such as art, when the future is so unknown. Even though there is a risk in creating, making art feels safe because it is known.
I am a reminder of your experiences and I will always be with you.	• I will never leave your mind. • I am a part of you. • I prove that everything happened. • I am a reminder of your strength. • I am a reminder that you survived. • I make you relive your experiences. • You lost everyone, but you have me.	Making art was necessary to remember every detail, and reminded artists that they had already gotten through so much. The art could serve as a reminder of people and places that no longer exist.
I affirmed your existence.	• I proved that you were there, even if you no longer exist. • I cast doubt on your existence. • You exist because of me. • I affirmed, declared, stated, swore, made factual, pledged, guaranteed, maintained your existence. • You will always exist because I exist. • In order to have disappeared, you had to first exist.	Artwork offered a sense of permanency—its tangible existence was permanent even if the individual's existence was not. It proved that the artist, and others, had lived in the world.

(Continued)

Table 7.2 Results of the phenomenological data analysis of the Holocaust artists *(Continued)*

Existential-phenomenological statement from the perspective of the artwork	*Imaginative variation*	*Summary statement of essence*
I gave you light.	• I am your only source of light. • Without me there is darkness. • Without me you have nothing. • All the light you have comes from me. • I remind you of light. • I help you remember light. • I am a reminder that lightness can exist. • You find light in me, remembering that it can exist.	Art served as a reminder that a sense of light was still possible, and therefore gave a sense of hope.
I keep you safe.	• I put you in danger. • I make you feel safe, even though you are not. • I allow you to overcome your fears. • If you are with me, then you are safe. • I let you feel safe. • I give an illusion of safety. • I let you transcend danger in order to feel safe.	There was a paradox in doing something danger-ous in order to feel safe. When making art, the artist could transcend danger and experience a brief sense of safety.
I gave you a purpose	• I was your purpose • I took away your purpose • I made you a purpose • I helped you find a purpose	Creating art provided hopeless victims with an increased sense of purpose.
I connect you to others	• I separated you from others • I introduced you to others • I secured bonds that once had • I am what bonds you to others • I am your only connection to those you love	Art making was often in service of or in response to other people. Art making was an act that connected the artist to someone they lost.

These results describe the phenomenon of art making within the Holocaust as a whole, without distinguishing the camp or ghetto of creation. Although the partic-ipants I interviewed described artistic activity in different settings, there were many overlaps in their descriptions of the experience. For example, Bak's narrative of art making in the Vilna ghetto resembled some aspects of Hošková-Weissová's reported experience. Milton (2000) found no geographical distinction in themes between eastern ghettos and concentration camps and western transit camps, noting the same categories across the artworks that developed in each separate location. This lack of differentiation further supports the overlapping experiences of art making I noticed in my interviews.

Additionally, though the experiences of individual artists were all unique, they could at least appreciate each other's motivation. In talking with Samuel Bak, it was clear that his motivation to make art in the Vilna ghetto was to provide a sense of hope to his community, to gain a sense of connection and to concretize his identity as an artist. This was what the art-making process offered to him. However, in our con-versation, he reflected on other artists who made clandestine art in the ghetto and understood how the process allowed them to document their situation and maintain a sense of humanity:

> If a very tired, poor artist in the ghetto is coming from digging some turf, comes back to the ghetto with his friend and says to his friend, "I know it's midnight but will you mind to sit there for a moment? I want to make a drawing of you." And if he makes a little drawing, a portrait of a tired man and so on, it helps him, of course, to find in himself something human. And he creates a document that tells this story (S. Bak, personal communication, October 10, 2017).

Bak's reason for creating art in the ghetto grew out of his individual needs, interests and lived experience as a nine-year-old trying to make sense of an incomprehensible situation. Having survived a ghetto and labor camp, decades later he could reflect on how other artists were motivated to document their existence and bolster their sense of humanity. Although the motivation behind his artwork differed from that of others, he recognized what motivated the artistic impulse of others. Because of this shared understanding and appreciation, I felt more confident in my results.

DISCUSSION

The results of my study suggest that the artists in this sample who created art during captivity in the Holocaust were motivated by the need to serve as a witness, to leave a legacy and to retain a sense of humanity. The experience offered a reinforcement of a non-prisoner identity; an affirmation of existence; a sense of hope; a sense of purpose; a feeling of safety; and an ability to develop, strengthen or embody relationships. These artists found comfort in doing something familiar amid deep uncertainty. Although creating often involved great risk, the actual process of making art felt safe and allowed artists to momentarily transcend the danger that surrounded them. Artwork offered a sense of permanence: its tangible substance felt permanent even as the artist's existence was not. It proved that the artist, and others, had existed in the world. The artwork itself ultimately became a reminder of what those targeted by Nazi oppression endured. It validated the resilience of these individuals in the face of cruelty and provided a sense of meaning within suffering. If, as Hinz (2017) articulated, creativity is a human right, engaging in creativity allowed these Holocaust survivors to remain human in even the most dehumanizing of environments.

The psychological structure that I found to describe the essence of the phenomenon of creating artwork in a concentration camp or ghetto is constructed from the elements of witnessing; identity; affirmation of existence; comfort; autonomy; connection; and hope. In the following paragraphs, I elaborate on each of these elements as they arose in my interviews.

Witnessing

The deep need to serve as a witness was a common motivator for these and other artists creating in captivity across Europe. Yehuda Bacon explained: "I wanted to be a witness. I was a child, and I thought, 'What can I do? I have to be a spokesman for the children's soul which does not exist anymore'" (Y. Bacon, personal communication, September 26, 2017). Bacon also referenced artists in the Terezín design department who utilized their access to art materials to clandestinely depict the horrors of life in Terezín, stating that those artists "wanted to give a witness into what [was] really happening. They had the same desire as me—'We must tell'—even though they paid with their life" (Y. Bacon, personal communication, September 26, 2017). Alon recalled a quote from Halina, her mother: "My observation, my need to observe what was going on, was stronger than my body. It was a need, a driving need" (as cited in Rosenberg, 2001, para. 6). This need to serve as a witness is congruent with Leclerc's (2011) findings that the role of witness was critical for Holocaust artists. Bak described his actual artwork as a witness, considering how the *Pinkus*—the book that he drew in—would take in the incomprehensible scenes: "German soldiers are dragging Father to the place of his execution. I am far away but I imagine the Pinkus witnessing the scene with its nonexistent eyes" (2001, p. 12)

Comfort

Few comforts were offered in either camps or ghettos. Although the act of making art was inherently unsafe, a feeling of safety emerged in the routine of drawing or painting. Jacobs recalled that her mother's desire to comfort children in Bergen-Belsen led her to organize art classes—"it was something that she knew how to do" (J. Jacobs, personal communication, September 1, 2017)—suggesting that her mother also benefited from the comfort of doing something familiar. Alice Ehrmann Shek found comfort by drawing secretly in the attic of her building, losing herself in her artwork. Alon expanded on this notion in relation to her own mother's drawing process: "You are doing something, so you must do that, not because you chose, not because you want, because you must. And if you stop, everything falls apart." She emphasized that when her mother was drawing, "nothing could happen to her" (M. Alon, personal communication, September 25, 2017). The content of Olomucki's works also reflects a sense of comfort: she repeatedly drew mothers embracing their children and women holding each other for warmth (Figures 7.1 and 7.2).

Hope

Although the environments in which these artists created were bleak, some artists found that drawing instilled a sense of hope. Jacobs recalled: "I had always loved butterflies and flowers. I think they were symbols of beautiful things you couldn't have in the camp. So drawing them reminded the kids that they could have hope" (J. Jacobs, personal communication, September 1, 2017). She elaborated that art was a mechanism for lifting morale, which made the children feel better about themselves: "In a sense it allowed for transcendence; it transported us out of this misery, at least temporarily" (J. Jacobs, personal communication, September 1, 2017).

While interned in the Vilna Ghetto at age nine, Bak sketched a portrait of Moses (Figure 6.3), which he later attempted to sculpt out of clay. He recalled his goal of displaying the image of Moses in the center of the ghetto, to remind all residents that the Jewish people had previously suffered persecution and were ultimately saved. "I knew that Moses was the great liberator of enslaved and oppressed Jews," Bak said, continuing, "It was he who led them out of Egypt, and therefore I figured that it would be very auspicious to create for the ghetto a sculpture in his honor" (2001, p. 18). Bak's drawing of Moses was an effort to remind his fellow ghetto residents to retain hope of salvation.

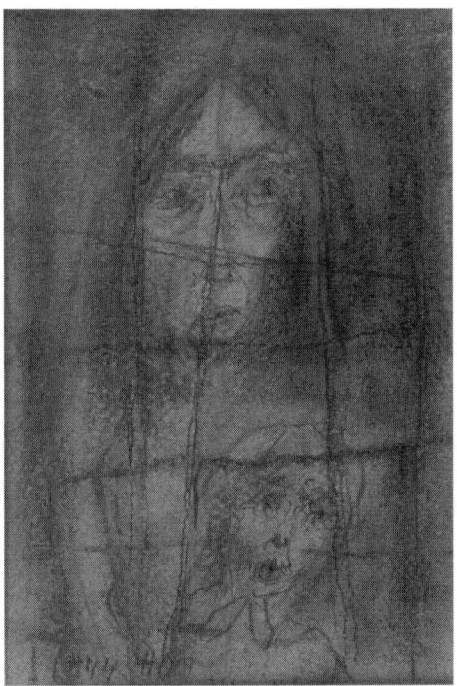

Figure 7.1 Halina Olomucki (1919–2007). *Mother and Child.* Poland, 1939–1945. Courtesy of the Ghetto Fighters' House Museum Art Collection, Western Galilee, Israel.

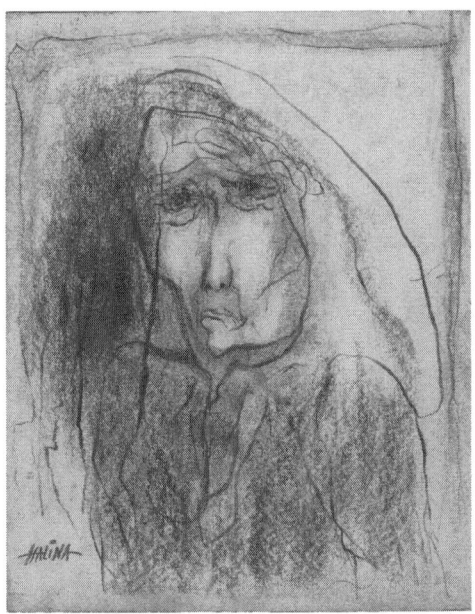

Figure 7.2 Halina Olomucki (1919–2007). *Woman in the Camp.* Auschwitz-Birkenau, 1943–1945. Courtesy of the United States Holocaust Memorial Museum.

Affirmation of Existence

Existence in camps and ghettos was tenuous and, according to Frankl (1973), "underwent a deformation" (p. 93). Many people recalled the disorienting reality of witnessing fellow prisoners fall prey to death. Talking about his close friend, the young artist Peter Ginz, Bacon stated:

> I saw him marching to the gas chamber. I was in Auschwitz and I knew exactly who would go to the gas chambers. I knew him and I saw him—I couldn't speak to him, it was forbidden—but I saw him with other children marching (Y. Bacon, personal communication, September 26, 2017).

Art making served as an affirmation of the artists' existence and concrete proof that they had survived another day. Alon reported that fellow inmates begged her mother, Halina, to paint their portraits "so that people won't forget them" (M. Alon, personal communication, September 25, 2017). When the line between life and death was precarious, art making affirmed that the artist, and those around them, had existed. As Bak (2001) described: "genuine artists tried in the bleakest of times to reassure themselves of their humanity and give value to their existence" (p. 20). In retrospect, Bak wondered if the poets who gave him a book to draw in had this intention:

> When they gave the book to me, they had some thoughts that at that age I wasn't able to grasp. That, "Maybe this child is condemned to death and he will not survive; maybe what he has to give, within the limits of what he can create, this will remain" (S. Bak, personal communication, October 10, 2017).

I noticed this theme in a document I read recently about the Polish artist Józef Szajna. Szajna survived Auschwitz and Buchenwald, and went on to study at the Academy of Art in Kraków. He is known for creating instillations and theater productions in response to his experience in these camps (Howard & Łubienski, 1989). His body of post-war art echoes this sentiment of affirmation. Though his artistic career began years after his liberation, his motivation was similar to those who made art in captivity: "I would consider myself immoral if I did not remember people who were murdered while I am here, alive" (as cited in Feinstein, 2000, p. 115). In creating artwork retrospectively, Szajna aimed to affirm the existence of those whom he suffered with.

Autonomy

Engelking (2005) described how prisoners in camps and ghettos lived under totalitarian oppression that resulted in a lack of choice or decision making in almost all aspects of their existence. Creating art, however, provided a unique opportunity to experience some degree of autonomy. Jacobs shared that by engaging children in art lessons, her mother "felt that if she could distract them and lift the morale, then she would have accomplished something" (J. Jacobs, personal communication, September 1, 2017). Frederick Terna explicitly described the sense of autonomy he felt by drawing:

> If one's life is sort of in a straitjacket of a concentration camp, with all the restrictions, well, a white sheet of paper and a drawing tool, there I am in control… that gave me an autonomy. That was what was pushing me, not the outside world (F. Terna, personal communication, September 5, 2017).

In our conversation, Thomas Geve also commented that drawing gave him a sense of control that he would not have otherwise felt during his time in Auschwitz (T. Geve, personal communication, November 9, 2020). By creating art, prisoners were able to exert a semblance of control in their mostly bound existence.

Identity

The importance of identifying as an artist was pervasive throughout this study. Bak spoke about his reputation as a talented nine-year-old artist in the Vilna ghetto. Rather than describing himself as a victim or a weak helpless child, Bak repeatedly called himself "a little prodigy" (S. Bak, personal communication, October 10, 2017). Alon described her mother's identity as an artist, saying, "It was such a big part of her." She elaborated: "Without that, she would have to find another way; but it was such a big part of her identity that if she didn't draw, she would lose herself. It wasn't a part of her; it was her" (M. Alon, personal communication, September 25, 2017). Remaining active in one's artist identity reminded Holocaust survivors that they served a purpose and allowed them to find meaning.

In some instances, art making provided individuals with a new identity. Terna explained that he never considered himself an artist prior to drawing in Terezín, but decided: "This is what I do, and if I survive, I will probably become an artist" (F. Terna, personal communication, September 5, 2017). When everything he knew had been destroyed, Terna used art to create a new reality for himself. Even at age 95, Terna continues to paint and exhibit his work.

The artists in this study described benefiting from the creation of artwork during the Holocaust. Although their situation was extreme, the benefits they derived from art making may resonate with or support contemporary art therapy practices. Bak explained: "Everything was amplified, so the artistic ego was amplified. This is how it was, the existence within the terribly destructive reality of the ghetto. It was somehow ruled by impulses that people also had in normal life" (S. Bak, personal communication, October 10, 2017). Bak's words suggest that the psychological needs of fellow prisoners became heightened, radical versions of their needs prior to captivity. Contemporary consumers of art therapy also need to bear witness; to gain hope; to feel that their existence is affirmed; to find comfort; to feel secure in their sense of identity; and to experience autonomy. If art making offered these benefits to individuals in extreme trauma and life-threatening conditions, then it can certainly support the myriad needs of individuals suffering today.

All but one of the artists detailed in the last chapter continued to make art well after liberation. Bak, a professional artist, stated that "my art therapy is my work. And I think that doing art is for many artists a therapy" (S. Bak, personal communication, October 10, 2017.) Terna concluded our interview by saying that he is an artist who "lives with the past and deals with it" through art (F. Terna, personal communication, September 5, 2017). Hošková-Weissová noted that her artwork is different now, but "it always goes back to the Holocaust" (H. Hošková-Weissová, personal communication, January 22, 2021).

Connection

The act of making art appeared to help artists build connections in an inherently lonely environment. This seemed especially important as many of the artists had been ostracized by their communities prior to their deportation and longed for a sense of belonging. Frederick Terna and Yehuda Bacon each mentioned the opportunities they had to share their drawings with well-known artists in Terezín, thus forming a new connection. The feedback from these artists—including Bedrich Fritta, Otto Ungar and Karel Fleishmann—gave them a sense of confidence in their artistic abilities and ultimately themselves. Being invited to join adult artists in the Vilna ghetto also served as a form of connection for Samuel Bak, as he began to establish relationships outside of his family. The acknowledgment that Terna, Bacon and Bak received from adult artists facilitated a new connection both with people whom they admired and with their artistic identity.

For Halina Olomucki, drawing connected her to other women in Birkenau. After losing her mother at the *Umschlagplatz* in Warsaw, Olomucki was completely separated from her family. She developed relationships with other women in Birkenau by drawing portraits for them upon request. This act of witnessing and capturing the likeness of other women, and the appreciation that they felt in return, strengthened the bond between artist and subject.

In other instances, art making was guided by a desire to remain connected to others who were not present with the artist. Thomas Geve and Helga Hošková-Weissová both described being motivated by their fathers. Geve wanted to bring something to his father when they were eventually reunited. He drew scenes from Auschwitz to have something tangible to give his father. Hošková-Weissová diligently drew what she observed in Terezín upon her father's suggestion to "draw what you see." Although both artists had been physically separated from their fathers, they maintained a connection to their fathers through their art.

LIMITATIONS

There were a number of limitations to this study, including the small sample size and the need to rely on narrative memory to recall events that happened decades ago. I could not directly observe the phenomenon I was researching, as it had occurred 70 years earlier. Thus, I could only rely on participants' accounts of the phenomenon. Moreover, I observed that the interviews cued the participants to share well-rehearsed stories of their experience. Even though they were comfortable divulging these stories, they clearly did so in a rote manner. I recognized certain phrases in my interviews that I had heard participants say before, almost verbatim, in documentaries and testimonies.

This discrepancy required me to more carefully qualify the study results by taking into account the distinction between lived experience and both the memory and the narrating of that lived experience as told, retold and elaborated over time. For example, while searching the literature, I came across a vignette about Yehuda Bacon saving his potato rations in Auschwitz to create a stamping tool. I brought this up when I first contacted Bacon and he responded with laughter. He insisted that had never happened and explained that stories from survivors can be altered and embellished as they are passed along anecdotally. He requested we meet in person so that I could hear his story directly from him, without any secondary distortions or embellishments.

Miriam Alon, the daughter of Halina Olumucki, reported that some of her mother's stories and written notes differed slightly from those of the Yad Vashem archives—a discrepancy Alon assumed was the result of historians attempting to make sense of confusing, fragmented, and inconsistent documentation. The validity of data and its generalization are two issues that Holocaust scholar Tec (2000) discussed in relation to the discrepancies that may present in accounts that are constructed from survivor memory. Tec argued that is impossible to make generalizations about Holocaust experiences from the memories of a sample of survivors, given that there are millions of accounts that perished in the Holocaust and therefore cannot be accessed or used to verify those of survivors. As Mieczysław Kościelniak stated in a testimony, "The handful of people who were allowed to make artistic works were only a fraction of a percent of those who suffered and died in Auschwitz. And how many eminent artists were among the dying".

Due to the serious implications of any research (as cited in Sieradzka, 2019) that involves experiences of the Holocaust, it is worth elaborating further on this point. Tec (2000) explained that the lapse in time since the Holocaust makes it difficult for survivors to accurately reconstruct chronological events. Tec noted that it is especially difficult for those who were children during the Holocaust to recount specifics such as dates and chronology of events. Furthermore, the samples of testimony that scholars do have access to represent only those individuals who survived and are able to share; the experiences of others—such as those who perished or who choose not to disclose their accounts—are both vast and inaccessible. Thus, it must be noted that these latter accounts actually make up a minority of the total victim experience and therefore cannot be used to form generalizations about the Holocaust.

As Tec's (2000) explication makes clear, the details of some of the experiences reported by participants in this study may contain information that is potentially different from what has been documented in other sources. In order to ensure that the information I received and ultimately presented was accurate, I stepped out of the phenomenological method and searched archival information to corroborate my findings. I was able to listen to recordings of verbal testimonies that some of the participants had given to substantiate my interviews. I also found archival information on specific aspects that the participants had mentioned, such as the Auschwitz family camp, the *Umschlagplatz* and the *aktions* in the Vilna ghetto. Ultimately, the results in this text serve to present phenomenological elements that were synthesized from descriptive data directly provided by the participants. I have successfully corroborated dates and locations from these narrative accounts with archival sources.

Another limitation of the study was the unavoidable subjectivity I experienced when engaging with my participants. Although I attempted to bracket off information that I already knew about each individual and their circumstances, it was difficult to bracket off what I had previously read about their lives. As previously stated, I became interested in this body of Holocaust artwork through having seen it personally. The artwork left a powerful imprint in my mind; and although that imprint motivated my research, it also hindered my ability to fully adopt the phenomenological attitude. Due to the power of the subject matter, I could not fully bracket off what I already knew about the Holocaust, the artwork made and what I had previously read about my participants.

My subjectivity to this research also came from my identity as a Jewish artist. I related to my participants on a religious, cultural and artistic level. I recognized that had I lived in Europe during WWII, I also would have been targeted. I reflected on this during my trip to Berlin. After seeing the exhibit *Art from the Holocaust* and attending a related lecture, I walked through the city to get dinner. I felt completely safe walking in an unfamiliar area and took my time to appreciate the sunset and views. It occurred to me that just 70 years prior, I would not have had that luxury. Someone in my position—perhaps even the artists whose work I had just seen—would be unable to safely make that exact walk. A lone Jewish woman in Hitler's Germany would avoid the walk due to fear of being accosted, assaulted or arrested; while I enjoyed a leisurely experience. While I appreciated how much had changed in those 70 years, it was impossible to remove myself from the history of my setting. This memory parlayed into my research, making me feel even closer to the participants.

Upon reviewing my transcripts, the rehearsed nature of the participants' interviews stood out to me. The survivors I interviewed are willing to share their stories and have done so many times, primarily in educational settings. In contrast, according to a curator at the United States Holocaust Museum and Memorial, the topic of the Holocaust evokes for the general public memories of black and white photos of walking corpses in striped uniforms (K. Schuster, personal communication, 2018) and similar horrifying imagery. Given these images, it is unsurprising that people often listen to survivors' tales with an expectation that the most gruesome details of their story will be included. Although the survivors have been free for decades, they are continually asked to detail the most dehumanizing experience of their lives. Their story is often flattened to one of starvation, hurt and loss. The nuances of their account can get lost in favor of a sensationalized account of how they defied death.

In his writings on interpreting the narratives of Holocaust survivors, Greenspan (1999) noted the difference between tragedy and atrocity, and how that discrepancy makes survivors' stories difficult both to tell and to hear. He explained that the Holocaust as a whole is taught, and therefore conceptualized, as an atrocity, characterized by mass death and degradation. Greenspan classified survivors' narratives as tragedies, marked by a smaller number of individuals and a more structured sequence of events. He stated: "in tragedy victims are still identifiably living and human, not atrocity's doomed, defeated, or walking dead" (Greenspan, 1999, p. 87).

The problem lies in how a survivor shares their tragedy as immersed in an atrocity. How can they tell what happened specifically to them when there is so much more to the story as a whole? I surmise that some survivors have become accustomed to the expectations of their listeners and therefore have structured their narratives in such a way that their unique experience both is conveyed and matches the publicly familiar context of the Holocaust as atrocity.

The horrific details are critical to Holocaust education because the mass scale of the atrocity must be fully expressed. However, the atrocity of the Holocaust is made up of millions of individual tragedies that can get lost in the overwhelming numbers of death and destruction. Greenspan (1999) quoted a survivor he has interviewed multiple times about witnessing one man's death in a work camp and how that experience differed from what the survivor had witnessed later in an extermination camp:

> People hadn't become ciphers yet. They were still, up to that moment, human beings. With a name, with a personality. And when they were gone, their image was retained.

> But the mass disappearing into the gas chambers – they're just a mass of people going, like in a slaughterhouse (p. 87).

The individual stories of survivors can be seen as atypical of what is expected from Holocaust testimony (Greenspan, 1999), since the focus is on the few rather than the masses. The human qualities of the individuals are overshadowed and often do not fit what is envisaged about the Holocaust. But these individual tragedies are what is so imperative for Holocaust education, as they are accessible and relatable, and can ultimately evoke compassion and empathy. The diary of Anne Frank is an example of this: situated within the Holocaust, it tells the story of one family from an adolescent girl's perspective. Readers can relate to and feel genuine compassion for the Frank family because the perspective is narrow and, to an extent, familiar. Exposure to individual accounts of the Holocaust can potentially enhance understanding and empathy, as these smaller-scale stories are easier to comprehend than mass extermination.

Because my study centered on the unique experience of art making in Nazi camps and ghettos, I sought out these individual stories. Inquiring about their artwork, I invited participants to share their distinct stories from their exclusive perspective as both artist and survivor. I did not regard them as nameless victims who were indistinguishable from the masses, but as artists. They were able to talk about what humanized, rather than dehumanized, them. I did not ask follow-up questions about the Holocaust as a whole, but limited the focus to their experience creating art, which made space for their individual story to be emphasized. The 94-year-old Frederick Terna eagerly walked up the three flights of stairs in his home to his studio to expound on how he had improvised brushes and pens in Terezín. He pointed out the jars of sand he collects to add texture to his work, as dirt and sand were the only materials he could access in the Kaufering work camp. He commented that he was glad we met in his home so that he could demonstrate how he had managed to make his art in Terezín.

I was grateful to be in Terna's presence and to absorb all that he was willing to share. I was struck by how committed he was to making his artwork in the ghetto and how that commitment has stayed with him throughout his life. Terna seemed genuinely excited to share his process with me, which was a response to my genuine interest in learning about it. The materials and techniques he used in Terezín, as well as the other artists who influenced him, are not just part of his captivity, but make up his identity as an artist. During his time in Terezín, his artistic identity helped to humanize him. In showing me his studio and materials, Terna conveyed himself not just as a Holocaust survivor, but as an artist. Terna, and the other artists I interviewed were able to maintain a sense of humanity despite their dehumanizing circumstances. By interviewing participants about their art, rather than limiting our discussion to their suffering, I encouraged them to share one of the few, but major, humanizing aspects of their experience that has shaped their identity to this day.

In reflecting on this study, I am keenly aware of the limitations that I faced. I wanted to understand the phenomenon of making art within the Holocaust; but due to the massive data that qualitative research produces, I was limited to a small sample. Because over 340,000 works of artwork have been documented from the Holocaust, it would be impossible to describe the essence of the phenomenon from just eight accounts. Additionally, the passage of time can distort one's memory and narration of events, making some aspects of the survivors' accounts potentially contestable.

What I was able to do, however, was to verify the results of my study against what has been documented and discussed in the literature. The psychological statement of essence that I arrived at was consistent with the writings of Holocaust art scholars (Bohm-Duchen, 2013; Moreh-Rosenberg, 2016). Conversations I had with curators at Yad Vashem, the United States Holocaust Memorial Museum and Beit Terezín, as well as Holocaust art scholars Elena Marakova and Giedrė Jankevičiūtė, also supported my results. Both Yehuda Bacon and Frederick Terna mentioned interactions with the artists in the Terezín design department, including Leo Haas and Bedrich Fritta, whose accounts are heavily documented in Holocaust art literature (Green, 1978; Blatter & Milton, 1981; Costanza, 1982). Bacon and Terna's interactions were consistent with the literature and this consistency supported the validity of my claims. While it is impossible to make any generalizations about the Holocaust from a small sample comprised exclusively of survivors narrating their accounts from decades ago (Tec, 2000), I can say that the phenomenological themes I identified were corroborated by literature and findings of other Holocaust art scholars.

CONCLUSIONS

The artists who participated in this study had suffered through different camps and ghettos across Europe, but shared similar experiences of art making in captivity. Engaging in artistic pursuits did not guarantee survival and in some instances hindered it. However, art making did benefit the artists in some capacity and perhaps made their abysmal reality more bearable. By creating artwork while in captivity, these artists were able to affirm their sense of existence; retain a sense of identity; gain a degree of hope, comfort and autonomy; and serve as a witness for those who perished. By exploring the experience of art making for those in desperate need of healing almost a century ago, we can understand how art making led to psychic survival when one's very existence was untenable. In the following section, I will detail theories that align with this theme of psychic survival to show how the art from the Holocaust illustrates the finding of meaning within an experience of suffering.

REFERENCES

Bak, S. (2001). *Painted in words*. Bloomington, IN: Indiana University Press.

Blatner, J. & Milton, S. (1981). *Art of the Holocaust*. New York, NY: Routledge.

Bohm-Duchen, M. (2013). Creativity against all odds: Art and internment during World War II. In P. Tame, D. Jeannerod, & M. Braganca (eds.). *Mnemosyne and Mars: Artistic and cultural representations of twentieth-century Europe at war* (pp. 183–201). London, England: Cambridge Scholars.

Costanza, M. (1982). *The living witness: Art in the concentration camps and ghettos*. New York, NY: The Free Press.

Engelking, B. (2005). *Holocaust and memory*. New York, NY: A&C Black.

Feinstein, S. (2000). Art after Auschwitz: Jozef Szajna's "Theater of Panic". In F. C. DeCoste and B. Schwartz (eds.). *The Holocaust's ghost: Writings on art, politics, law and education*. Edmonton, AB: University of Alberta Press, 109–123.

Finlay, L. (1999). Applying phenomenology in research: Problems, principles and practice. *British Journal of Occupational Therapy, 62*(7), 299–306. doi: 10.1177/030802269906200705

Finlay, L. (2011). *Phenomenology for therapists: Researching the lived world.* Hoboken, NJ: John Wiley & Sons.

Frankl, V. E. (1973). *The doctor and the soul: From psychotherapy to logotherapy* (R. Winston & C. Winston, trans.). New York, NY: Vintage Books. (Original work published 1946.)

Giorgi, A. (2009). *The descriptive phenomenological method in psychology: A modified Husserlian approach.* Pittsburgh, PA: Duquesne University Press.

Giorgi, A. (2012). The descriptive phenomenological psychological method. *Journal of Phenomenological Psychology, 43*(1), 3–12. doi: 10.1163/156916212x632934

Giorgi, A. & Giorgi, B. (2003). The descriptive phenomenological psychological method. In P. M. Camic, J. E. Rhodes & L. Yardley (eds.). *Qualitative research in psychology: Expanding perspectives in methodology and design.* Washington, DC: American Psychological Association, pp. 243–273.

Green, G. (1978). *The artists of Terezin.* New York, NY: Hawthorn Books.

Greenspan, H. (1999). Listening to Holocaust survivors: Interpreting a repeated story. *Shofar: An Interdisciplinary Journal of Jewish Studies, 17*(4), 83–88.

Hinz, L. D. (2017). The ethics of art therapy: Promoting creativity as a force for positive change. *Art Therapy, 34*(3), 142–145. doi: 10.1080/07421656.2017.1343073

Howard, T, & Łubienski, T. (1989). The theatres of Józef Szajna. *New Theatre Quarterly, 5*(19), 240–263.

Kapitan, L. (2018). *Introduction to art therapy research.* New York, NY: Routledge.

Leclerc, J. (2011). Re-presenting trauma: The witness function in the art of the Holocaust. *Art Therapy, 28*(2), 82–89. doi: 10.1080/07421656.2011.580181

Moreh-Rosenberg, E. (2016). *The art from the Holocaust.* Cologne, Germany: Wienand Verlag.

Rosenberg, P. (2001). *Learning about the Holocaust through art.* http://art.holocaust-education.net/

Tec, N. (2000). Diaries and oral history: Some methodological considerations. *Religion and the Arts, 4*(1), 87–95.

PART 3
PRACTICE

My first job out of graduate school was as an art therapist on an inpatient eating disorders unit within a large behavioral health system. Art therapy had long been a major component of the unit's programing and was considered a valued element of patient treatment. I worked with patients primarily in groups and occasionally individually, and was able to share their artworks in daily rounds with an interdisciplinary staff. In these meetings, I noticed that my patient reports, including their artwork, were different from those of my counterparts in other disciplines. Although the psychiatrist, family therapist and psychologist typically discussed the challenging aspects of our patients' illnesses, my reports often highlighted another side. The artworks I shared provided a depth of insight into the patient as a whole and beyond the parameters of their disorder. I felt that patients' engagement in art therapy illuminated a unique, unseen aspect of them that was often eclipsed by their illness. Art making seemed to ignite their spirit and their artwork invited me to experience them more fully.

This realization that patient artwork can uniquely elucidate the humanness of an individual was in part informed by exposure to artwork created by those targeted by Nazi oppression during the Holocaust. As I mentioned previously, I had first learned about the phenomenon of Holocaust artwork right as I was beginning formal art therapy training. The concept behind this phenomenon—that individuals were able to retain a sense of identity and humanness through art making—has shaped my own practice of art therapy.

I had hoped that the research process I detailed in Part 2 of this text would further inform my art therapy practice. My findings indicated that artists who created during the Holocaust did benefit from the art-making process and I have since reflected on whether contemporary art therapy clients might achieve a similar benefit. This is not to suggest that the experiences or needs of my clients are analogous to those of Holocaust victims. What I do propose is that if individuals in camps and ghettos were able to transcend their conditions to feel a sense of hope, comfort, autonomy and identity, then perhaps art therapy consumers, when led by an art therapist, could reap similar benefits. And likewise, perhaps art therapists could learn from the artists of the Holocaust to shift how they practice to a way that is focused on developing a greater sense of humanity within their clients. In the following chapters, I expound on how essential themes from the study of artists who created during the Holocaust are currently guiding my clinical work. I ground the phenomenon of Holocaust artwork in existential theory and logotherapy, a theoretical framework developed by Holocaust survivor Viktor Frankl. I believe that the search for meaning that is fundamental to logotherapy supports artists' motivation for creating during captivity. In the final chapter, I illustrate how logotherapy and my research inform my art therapy practice using case vignettes.

DOI: 10.4324/9781003160885-11

CHAPTER 8

GROUNDING THE ART OF THE HOLOCAUST IN THE PHILOSOPHIES OF EXISTENTIALISM AND LOGOTHERAPY

The findings from my phenomenological study of the Holocaust art phenomenon indicated that art making within a Nazi camp or ghetto yielded seven thematic results: witnessing; comfort; hope; affirmation of existence; autonomy; connection; and identity. These results were consistent with the literature on Holocaust artwork and I was able to confirm them again when I interviewed additional survivors and kin for this text. As I wanted to demonstrate that my research could inform art therapy practice, I sought to ground my findings in existing theory within psychology and art therapy literature. To do so, I considered what united these themes. The obvious connection to me was the existential construct of *meaning*. Each of these seven themes in some way contributed to a sense of meaning for the artist. I decided to look at meaning through the existential lens of Viktor Frankl, since his writings were heavily influenced by his own experiences in Terezín, Auschwitz, and Dachau.

I initially became acquainted with Frankl's philosophies when writing my master's thesis in 2008 on Freidl Dicker-Brandeis's work in Terezín. My advisor suggested I read Frankl's most famous book, *Man's Search for Meaning*, which was my first introduction to existentialism and logotherapy. There was a particular quote in the text that stood out to me in the context of Holocaust artwork:

> Those martyrs, whose behavior in camp, whose suffering and death, bore witness to the fact that the last inner freedom cannot be lost... It is this spiritual freedom, which cannot be taken away – that makes life meaningful and purposeful (2006, p. 67).

Frankl was not specifically referring to the artists of Terezín, Auschwitz or Gurs; though he could have been. The phrase "whose behavior in camp" resonated with Dissanayake's (1995) description of art as a *behavior*, which suggests that art is made instinctively for both pleasure and survival. Frankl's ideas of *spiritual freedom* and *meaning and purpose* helped me to understand Dicker-Brandeis's drive in Terezín and continued to resonate as I learned more about the phenomenon of Holocaust artwork over the next decade. I realized that my own practice had been shaped by these ideas, and that I needed to learn more about existential philosophy in order to better articulate how it related to both my research and practice.

As I dove into the field of existentialism, with the help of my mentor Bruce Moon, I noticed myriad ways in which the philosophy pertained to my research. Existentialism is a theory which has helped me to comprehend the art of the Holocaust not as images of trauma, but as a confrontation with the realities of a fleeting existence. In my clinical practice, existential theory has taught me how to see my clients beyond the pathology that they present. Although Part 3 of this text is built around practice, I must first elaborate on existential theory and its successor, logotherapy, for the reader to better elucidate the connection I have made between these theories and Holocaust artwork.

While writing this text, I was put in touch with Alex Vesely Frankl, grandson of Viktor Frankl. Vesely Frankl is a trained logotherapist and founder of the

DOI: 10.4324/9781003160885-12

Viktor Frankl Institute of America, an organization dedicated to Frankl's philosophy and teaching. Vesely Frankl also sits on the board of the Viktor Frankl Institute in Vienna, which offers training programs in logotherapy and existential analysis. He has traveled the world lecturing on his grandfather's philosophy. He is also a director of Noetic Films, a Los Angeles-based studio that specializes in mental health-related content.

Vesely Frankl and I spoke about logotherapy via FaceTime and I have been able to consult with him on this text since our initial conversation regarding the nuances of his grandfather's philosophy. He has referenced conversations with his grandfather that have helped me better comprehend the philosophy of logotherapy—which, as he explained, is underdeveloped in North American literature. Our conversation was reminiscent of my interviews with second-generation Holocaust survivors, as I was learning about a philosophy through a narrative account. Alex described logotherapy with the same examples and analogies that his grandfather had used to teach him; and I valued this opportunity to discuss logotherapy one step removed from its creator. My descriptions of logotherapy in the ensuing paragraphs come from Frankl's writings (1967, 1973, 1988, 2004, 2006), as well as from conversations and correspondence with his grandson.

EXISTENTIALISM

The precarious balance of life and death in ghettos and camps forced victims to deeply contemplate their own existence. This is evident in survivor testimonies, victim journal entries and the artwork that was made in such environments. An embrace of existentialism, defined as the philosophical concern for human existence (Jones, 2001), became one response to the Holocaust by both surviving victims and scholars (Frankl, 2006; Levi, 1985). In fact, the existential psychotherapy movement gained momentum in the mid-1940s in part as a response to the global atrocities of WWII and the horrors of the Holocaust in particular. The elucidation of existentialism in Western psychotherapy provided a paradigm that helped psychotherapists understand their clients as whole beings apart from their pathology (van Deurzen, 2012). Influenced by early existential philosophers—such as Søren Kierkegaard, Friedrich Nietzsche, Martin Heidegger and Jean-Paul Sartre—modern existentialists considered the chaotic, transient and circumstantial nature of human existence, from which they challenged the axioms of conventional psychotherapy practice (May & Yalom, 2000). In addition to including a spiritual, humanistic element in therapy, they believed that a psychotherapy session was a place to explore and discuss the uncomfortable but relevant ultimate concerns of existence, such as death, freedom, isolation and meaninglessness (Yalom, 1980).

Freedom is a crucial component of existential therapy, particularly in how the therapist practices. Relevant literature suggests that through an existential orientation, the therapist aims to free the client from the assumptions of how one *should* exist within their relationships, environment and society. For example, Moon (2009) stated that: "existential therapists are dedicated to liberating humanity from its denial of inescapable anxieties, fears, and shallow routines" (p. 6). Schneider and Krug (2017) aim to "set clients free" (p. 37) in an existential-humanistic practice. And Yalom and Josselson (2014) described the goal in existentially oriented therapy as that of "rediscovering the living person amid the dehumanization of modern culture" (p. 272). These acts of freedom, liberation and rediscovery all point to the notion of inviting an individual to look beyond a culturally sanctioned view of how they *should* live to consider how they truly *want* to live. This act of freedom in existential therapy serves as an invitation to clients to consider the authenticity of their existence. My own existential practice encourages clients to liberate or free themselves from the construct of what they deem is appropriate to discuss, or draw, in therapy. I invite them to rediscover their authentic selves though an exploration of the deeper, potentially controversial thoughts they harbor with regard to their own existence.

Existential therapy does not provide answers, but invites clients to ask and reflect on their inner questions (Schneider & Krug, 2017). The focus in an existential therapy session is not on symptom amelioration or behavior analysis, but instead on facing the realities of how one engages—or wants to engage—in their world (Yalom & Josselson, 2014). Existential therapy promotes a confrontation with the fearful realities of clients' lives, beyond the psychiatric symptoms and negative behaviors that are of focus in other forms of psychotherapy. Yalom and Josselson (2014) expressed concern that the existential crisis of clients—literally, their concerns pertaining to existence—is "masked" (p. 266) by symptoms that lead to a formal psychiatric diagnosis. In affixing this label[1] to the client, the therapist can appease the requirements of the US healthcare system and can converse about the client with other clinicians; but this ultimately limits the depth of what can be explored in therapy. The existential psychotherapist strives to dialogue with the client, not their behaviors, guiding the client to understand their concerns as embedded in an increased awareness and genuine fear surrounding their own existence. In this model, anxieties are not idiosyncratic, but rather are viewed as universal to the human condition.

While many mainstream psychological approaches focus on the self, the existential approach values the experience of the individual in the context of their world (van Deurzen & Arnold-Baker, 2018). Anxieties and other psychological struggles are viewed as problems related to how one lives and how one exists within their environment. Existential theory recognizes that most struggles ultimately pertain to an individual's existence in the world. The goal in existentially oriented therapy is not to eradicate a problem, since problems are viewed as functions of existing as a human in society and are therefore impossible to fully dispose of. Instead, the existential therapist guides the client to respond to the problem in a new, constructive way (Schneider, 2015). Rather than offering techniques, existential therapy is an exploration and appreciation of human existence and related limitations (Schneider & Krug, 2010; Cooper, 2015; Sousa, 2015). Existential therapy cannot be understood through a manual (Hoffman, et al, 2014), but rather through interpersonal engagement (Schneider & Krug, 2010).

---

1   In saying this, I recognize that a formal diagnosis is often required for insurance coverage. And often clients present with a very obvious diagnosis. I don't completely admonish the use of diagnostic criteria, and in fact find it useful in helping clients, their families and other clinicians understand the severity and context of the client's suffering. However, in operating from an existential framework, it is imperative for the therapist not to limit their perception of the client to symptoms and behaviors. Doing so would neglect the human spark that must be ignited in order to heal.

This can be difficult to comprehend in the abstract, so I will share an innocuous example from my outpatient clinical practice to illustrate the concept. I share this to emphasize the philosophical and relational aspects of existential theory.

Many of my adolescent clients expressed fear and anxiety about returning to in-person learning as schools introduced hybrid models during the Covid-19 pandemic. This was especially prevalent during the late summer and early fall of 2021, when many students returned to the classroom in person for the first time in almost 18 months. Their fears ranged from feeling uncomfortable with how their body may have changed—as is common in adolescence—to anxiety around being in large groups, to a fear of socializing again. I started noticing overlaps from client to client and realized that this anxiety was not unique, but universal. Looking at these concerns through an existential lens, I saw that these teens had experienced a significant shift in their daily existence and did not know how they would return to normalcy. The convention of school had grounded their existence for over a decade, providing a sense of routine and organization that was turned upside down in March 2020. The daily interactions and social expectations that were part of school culture were put on hold while students learned virtually from laptops, often without any in-person contact or connection. As challenging as that shift was, students had acclimated. Suddenly, they were returning to the pre-pandemic conventional routine, but feared that they would not know how.

After hearing multiple clients describe this uncertainty about the return to school, I reflected on Moon's (2009) discussion of the internal void that he noticed in adolescent clients. This internal void, characterized by the lack of a sense of self, is the result of a severed foundation and loss of groundedness. For many of my clients, the structure of school provided a reliable foundation from which they could develop interests, skills and relationships. The traditions that shaped school life—such as sports, dances and other extracurricular activities—had been paused; and though my clients were eager to resume these traditions, they worried they didn't know how. Their sense of self in the context of the school environment had diminished. At the core of this fear was an uncertainty regarding how to exist and function in an environment that had once been so familiar.

I found it was helpful to invite my clients to view their anxieties through the existential paradigm. Their fears were not functions of a clinical diagnosis, but instead stemmed from the uncertainty of their own existence in relation to school. We discussed how their routines had been abruptly changed and were being changed again, and how their anxieties were appropriate responses to this shift in existence. I also shared that I was hearing the same concerns from most of my clients in that age group, to accentuate how common this fear had become. This shift in perspective from their anxiety being unique to universal seemed to help. They recognized that their fears were a response to a changing experience of existence that had become quite common during the global pandemic.

I did not provide set art directives for this discussion, but encouraged art making in response to what the client was saying. For example, in one session with a client who shared that she did not know how to navigate around the physical school building or the social dynamics of ninth grade, I suggested drawing a metaphorical path with all the uncertainties that she would encounter as potential hiccups. Another client drew a similar path, but added magazine images to represent the external factors that hindered her confidence. In both sessions, I asked the client to consider if any of their friends might be navigating a similar path, which led to a conversation about how everyone—even teachers—would be traversing this unknown course for the first time since the pandemic hit. In other sessions, I asked clients to depict their anxieties abstractly or metaphorically, in order to give them tangible form so that they could be recognized. Engaging in the art process while discussing the reintegration to school gave clients an additional space in which to place and reflect on their fears and anxieties. Creating artwork about their anxieties allowed them to better understand and then confront the uncertain feelings that were causing discomfort. For some, the art process itself was soothing and in turn a comfort, which made the discussion feel safer.

YALOM'S FOUR CONCERNS OF EXISTENCE

The philosophical roots of existentialism suggest a favor to intellectualism (Van Deurzen, 2007), giving it a reputation for seeming unapproachable and elitist. However, at its core, existentialism is centered on the very basic experience of being in the world—something that all humans encounter. Yalom's (1980) take on existential psychotherapy helps to challenge the overly philosophical assumptions about existentialism and make the theory more accessible and applicable to daily life. Psychiatrist Irving Yalom articulated a clear relationship between existential philosophy and psychotherapy practice, which is rooted in European and Western philosophy. Yalom's (1980) theory centers on four primary concerns pertaining to existence: death, freedom, isolation and meaninglessness. These "givens," he asserted, shape human experience and encompass the deepest levels of existence. Any psychological struggle can be stripped down to one of these primary concerns, as they are all part of the human condition.

Although Yalom's four concerns were conceptualized for psychotherapy practice, the fact that they encapsulate the fundamental experiences of existence makes them relevant to an understanding of Holocaust victims in the context of their suffering. Having been forcibly removed from their pre-war lives to witness senseless violence and murder, Holocaust victims found their existence stripped down to these same core concerns; which is precisely why I have grounded my understanding of Holocaust artwork in existential theory. To highlight this connection, in the following paragraphs I elaborate on Yalom's existential givens with examples from my study on Holocaust art.

Death

The fear of death is paramount in Yalom's theory. He alleged that humans are naturally afraid of death, which is manifested as a death anxiety (Yalom, 2008). Like his predecessors, Yalom believed that most neuroses stem from a trepidation of human mortality that causes people to ignore or deny the subject completely. Instead, Yalom advised a confrontation with the inevitable, stating: "we should contemplate our ultimate end, familiarize ourselves with it, dissect and analyze it, reason with it, and discard terrifying childhood death distortions" (2008, p. 276). Existentialism views the definitiveness of life and death as interchangeable, thereby making the subject of death a critical topic in psychotherapy. If an individual can accept their ultimate fate, Yalom argued, they can live a more authentic life. Acknowledging that death is inevitable gives humans the opportunity to fully appreciate the life they have.

Yalom encourages a confrontation with the unsettling, often unpleasant realities of life, including death. The act of confrontation explicitly links existential theory to the art of the Holocaust, as artists confronted their disturbing realities in their artwork. This is most apparent in artworks that literally show death, through either a single corpse or a pile of bodies. In drawing images of death, artists confronted it and acknowledged it as part of their reality.

Marianne Grant was shocked at the piles of bodies she saw in Bergen-Belsen, to which she was evacuated from Auschwitz in 1945. She instinctively began to draw them in an attempt to make sense of the atrocity that continued to stun her (Grant, 2002). Zoran Music's series of corpses from Dachau differs, in that he had the experience of watching many of his subjects die. In an explanation to a liberation doctor, he stated: "I started drawing one man who was so far gone that he was dead by the time I finished the sketch" (as cited in Smith, 1972, pp. 84-85). His work does not confront the mass deaths, but instead explores the fine line between life and death. Amish Maisals (1993) noted that Music's drawings "convey the feeling that that these people had been alive just moments ago" (p. 52).

Some scholars have critiqued these brutal artworks for sensationalizing violence. Adorno argued that "there is something disagreeable, almost dishonorable, in the conversion of the suffering of the victims into works of art which are then thrown as fodder to the world that murdered them" (as cited in Hanson, 2006, p. 197). While this argument holds merit in the conversation of art and photographs of outside observers, I believe it is unfair to project this opinion onto the victims who lived alongside the subjects of these disturbing images. Death was very much part of their existence and their impetus to depict it suggests a confrontation with their reality. Their drawings appear to have been created in an attempt to confront the fragility of existence within the camps.

Freedom

Yalom's second concern, freedom, relates to Frankl's (1973) notion of free will and responsibility. Yalom believed that humans are responsible for their lives, their actions and their failures to act (1980). This concept of freedom is built on Sartre's (1949) theory of tension between authentic choice and ersatz comfort. Sartre asserted that humans have the freedom to live authentically, governed by their own moral compass. This freedom can cause anxiety when one senses "groundlessness" (Yalom, 1980) in the absence of firm external direction. The ability to act and to choose freely also involves a significant responsibility, which can contribute to anxiety or fear if experienced as overwhelming.

Although the individuals held captive in camps and ghettos were given very few freedoms, those who chose to create were able to exercise their freedom of choice. They chose how to live within the confines of their existence. This is exemplified in the artistic process of Franciszek Jaźwiecki, who, as I described in Chapter 3, drew portraits of fellow captives in Auschwitz and Buchenwald. Despite being severely punished when Nazi guards discovered his portraits, he resumed drawing. As a camp inmate, Jaźwiecki had very few freedoms. He knew that he would be reasonably safe if he stopped drawing and abided by the guards' orders. The fact that he was sent to a penal unit instead of to his death suggests that he was in good health and strong enough to potentially survive his captivity. The guards who administered his punishment likely saw that he was useful to them and worthy of life. Regardless of this, Jaźwiecki was an artist and found that his life was only worthwhile if he was able to draw. He knew the inherent risks, but chose to pursue the one freedom he could find. In continuing to draw, he chose authenticity over relative comfort. Jaźwiecki identified how he wanted to live within the parameters of camp life and made the choice to do so.

Isolation

Existential isolation refers to the recognition that no two people have an identical life experience. Each individual lives a completely unique existence in which they are solely responsible for their choices and actions. Yalom explained the concern of existential isolation as a breach in the human experience. Drawing on the works of Nietzsche, he wrote: "Each of us enters existence alone and must depart from it alone. The existential conflict is thus, the tension between our awareness of our absolute isolation and our wish to be part of a larger whole" (1980, p. 9). The concern of existential isolation is often experienced in individuals who are close to death, as they become acutely aware that they must die alone, and that their memory hinges on those who survive them. Yalom observed that the loss of a spouse can also trigger awareness of existential isolation, as the surviving spouse engages in their daily routines without the presence and observations of their life partner (Yalom & Josselson, 2004). The development of relationships throughout one's life may be a defense against existential isolation (May & Yalom, 2000).

I noticed this reconciliation with existential isolation in the artistic communities that developed in Terezín, Gurs, Vilnus, Ravensbrück, and Auschwitz. Many of the artists participating in these communities had been removed from their homes, families and communities, and undoubtedly recognized just how alone they truly were. The separation of these individuals from all that they knew of life reinforced the ultimate aloneness of their existence. Despite this stark realization, artists were able to find connectedness by engaging in art making together. Dicker-Brandeis, who could not bear a child of her own, created a legacy for herself by working with children in Terezín. Her actions allowed her to transcend the limits of her own life to touch and inspire the lives of others. Although her family name would not live on, her legacy did through her art lessons.

Female inmates at the Ravensbrück camp came from diverse backgrounds and yet found connection in their similarities. French resistance fighters, German political prisoners and young Jewish women joined together to draw, paint and craft— often in service of each other. They developed surrogate families in an effort to find connection, despite the inherent isolation they experienced. The artworks that they created for one another highlight this connectedness.

Meaninglessness

In his 1980 text, Yalom identified the existential concern of *meaninglessness*, which pertains to a void in the human experience. He used the term *meaning* in a more contemporary overview of existential psychotherapy (Yalom & Josselson, 2004), perhaps in an attempt to convey a more positive tone. Regardless of the wording, meaning is viewed by existentialists as a paramount concern. Yalom and Josselson explained that "one of our life tasks is to invent a purpose sturdy enough to support a life" (2004, p. 268). That is, the task of finding meaning in life is to identify what makes life worth living. Meaning is found when an individual engages in a fulfilling, self-transcending venture (Yalom & Josselson, 2004; Frankl, 1973). Meaninglessness— the absence of meaning—renders individuals purposeless and empty, ultimately leading to despair.

I believe that Holocaust artists found meaning through their practice of art making. Existence in a camp or ghetto was inherently meaningless. Individuals were cut off from the relationships, occupations and conventions that characterized their meaning prior to captivity. Many victims fell into despair and viewed their life as meaningless. The artists whom I have described in this text, however, defied the assumption of meaninglessness and found a reason to endure. Halina Olomucki, for example, who had been separated from her entire family, found meaning in commemorating the women around her in Birkenau. She explained:

> This need to document became an extraordinary force that carried me to survival. It became the foundation of my will power. My sole purpose in life was to live so I would be able to testify before the world about the most terrible of all atrocities and the courage of all the inmates of Auschwitz (as cited in Novitch, Dawidowicz & Freudenheim, 1981, pp. 17–18).

In drawing portraits, Olomucki identified a personal meaning that inspired her to endure.

Polish artist Xawery Dunikowski was imprisoned in Auschwitz for almost five years. After obtaining art materials in the infirmary in 1944, he stated that: "For the first time in four years I have once again begun to draw… life once again acquires meaning and purpose" (as cited in Amishai-Maisels, 1993, p. 4). Dunikowski, an accomplished sculptor prior to WWII, was able to find meaning through drawing. Despite all that he had endured and witnessed since his arrest in 1940, drawing made his life worth surviving for.

Yalom's existential concerns can be understood through examples of Holocaust artwork. In creating, these artists addressed the ultimate concerns of their tenuous existence. They confronted the reality of death that surrounded them and the isolation that became apparent. They took responsibility for their actions and engaged in free will, ultimately finding personal meaning to withstand their suffering.

FACING THE CONCERNS OF EXISTENCE

Schneider (2015) described the impact of a traumatic experience on one's existence. In the context of his discussion, Schneider uses the term *trauma* to mean a shock—a change in how an individual experiences their world. He explains that this shock disrupts the individual's sense of security, as well as their perceptions of themselves and the world around them: "It has a way of stripping bare this culturally sanctioned frame… exposing us to our foundationless depths" (2015, p. 21). These depths are comprised of Yalom's primary concerns of existence. When an individual experiences a shock in their life, shattering their sense of security, safety and identity in the context of the world, they are forced to confront the core concerns of existence.

I use Schneider's example of *trauma* with trepidation. As previously stated, I avoid categorizing the art of the Holocaust within a trauma framework. It goes without saying that victims endured a tremendous, unimaginable trauma. The degree of trauma experienced by victims during the Holocaust is incomparable to what most clinicians see in contemporary practices, and so looking at artwork from the Holocaust exclusively through a trauma lens would mitigate the magnitude of it. Seligman (1995) classified the Holocaust as a chronic life-threatening situation, in which victims' safety and integrity, self-image, security and value systems were all threatened. The collapse of these systems of security and world understanding go beyond the jargon of trauma literature. Victims experienced a complete upheaval of their whole lives. With their entire worldview in collapse, victims faced the deepest concerns of existence. Their struggles were not about the trauma of the situation, but rather about how the upheaval completely changed their experience of existence.

Since the concept of existence was a paramount concern in ghettos and camps, I believe existential philosophy, rather than a trauma lens, is critical to the discussion of Holocaust art. Understanding the existential needs of these artists helps us to better understand their motivation for creating artwork, despite the very real risks. The artists who created in the uncertain and abysmal environments of camps and ghettos grappled with the deepest concerns of existence. My description of the artworks in Chapters 2 and 3 showed a reconciliation with Yalom's existential concerns of death, isolation, freedom and meaninglessness. This body of work, and the motivation for creating it, can be understood when contextualized in existential theory. Through art making, victim artists explored and reconciled the concerns of existence that surrounded them. Victims were regularly forced to acknowledge the reality of death and their tenuous grasp on their own lives. They were forced into a position where freedom was almost non-existent and one of the few freedoms available was how to live in the most indeterminate of conditions. Many were isolated from their families and communities, and struggled to find a sense of meaning within their suffering. Kosiec (1989) explained the overarching themes of existence that unite the Auschwitz Museum's art collection:

> If one poses the question, what is it that welds the Oswiecim (Auschwitz) gallery, despite the diversity of its exhibits, into a single whole, the answer is this: the single and ever present theme in Oswiecim was death – death and its opposite, the will to survive, the desire for freedom. All the camp artists struggled with this consciously or instinctively, directly or indirectly, in all possible artistic themes and forms (p. 7).

As Kosiec makes clear, the commonality that permeates this body of artwork is an exploration of the depths of existence. And how could it not when existence, or the struggle to maintain existence, was the guiding force in victims' minds?

Schneider (2015) argued that the predominant question in existential therapy is: "How is one willing to live, in this remarkable moment, with this exceptional opportunity to encounter one's pain?" (p. 22). George and Park (2014) asserted that all humans strive for value in life. Through art making, the artists of the Holocaust found a way to live in a dangerous and uncertain environment, confront their own pain and attain a sense of value. Drawing was not how victims treated the symptoms of their trauma; it was how they endured their tenuous existence in a chronically unpredictable environment. The exploration of existence and the sense of meaning that this can offer are the crux of existential theory.

THE DEVELOPMENT OF LOGOTHERAPY

The existential focus on the human condition motivated Austrian physician Viktor Frankl, who expounded on the value of suffering in his auto-ethnographic memoir of Auschwitz, finding that a sense of meaning and purpose was life enhancing (1959, 2006). Frankl began exploring existential theory in psychotherapy in the 1920s while working in psychiatric clinics in Austria. He was concerned that psychiatry and psychology had become consumed by science and neglected an individual's spirituality. Frankl argued that psychotherapy must involve an individual's values (1973). To recognize these values, along with their spirit and sense of personal meaning, Frankl conceived of "logotherapy" as a "meaning-centered psychotherapy" (2006, p. 98), stemming from the Greek word *logos,* which implies reason or intent. He explained: "a psychotherapy which not only recognizes man's spirit, but actually starts from it may be termed logotherapy. In this connection, logos is intended to signify 'the spiritual' and beyond that 'the meaning'" (Frankl, 1986, xvii).

Frankl's concept of logotherapy relies on an individual's uniquely human ability to find meaning. The search for personal meaning is part of the logotherapeutic process. Meaning varies from person to person and is constructed by one's passions, choices, relationships and goals. To "find meaning" is to recognize these unique qualities and values, and to make choices in favor of them, regardless of the circumstances:

> Ultimately, man should not ask what the meaning of his life is, but rather he must recognize that it is *he* who is asked. In a word, each man is questioned by life; and he can only answer to life by *answering for* his own life; to life he can only respond by being responsible. Thus, logotherapy sees in responsibleness the very essence of human existence (Frankl, 2006, p. 109).

Frankl emphasized the responsibility of finding one's meaning. Meaning exists, but must be found. Therefore, personal responsibility—taking the responsibility to find one's meaning—is a key factor in logotherapy.

In addition to the term *logotherapy,* Frankl frequently referenced *existential analysis.* This term refers to the therapeutic process of a psychotherapist leading clients to an awareness of their capacity for meaning and finding the "hidden logos of [their] existence" (Frankl 1985a, p. 125). *Existential analysis* is therefore the practice of *logotherapy* and Frankl regularly used the two terms interchangeably. As many early art therapy programs were rooted in psychoanalytic theory, I will use the term *logotherapy* instead of *existential analysis,* to avoid confusion or misinterpretation of the concept. *Logotherapy* is also referred to as the *Third Viennese School of Psychotherapy,* following Freudian and Adlerian theory. Conceptualizing logotherapy as a separate school of thought further helps to distinguish it as its own entity.

Frankl earned fame throughout Europe before and during WWII for his compassionate treatment of patients and his critique of reductionism in psychiatric and medical practice (Längle & Sykes, 2006). As a director in a Jewish psychiatric hospital in Vienna, he bravely falsified the diagnoses of patients to save them from Nazi-enforced euthanasia. Frankl's first manuscript, *The Doctor and the Soul,* accompanied him to Terezín and later to Auschwitz. His wife sewed the papers into his coat in hopes of preserving them. Although the manuscript did not survive, Frankl and his philosophy did. In Terezín, he organized a "mental hygiene clinic" for ghetto residents, demonstrating his commitment both to humanity and to his own life's meaning, which he already considered paramount to existence.

In Auschwitz, Frankl's hope and optimism that he would one day be reunited with his wife contributed to his psychic survival (Frankl, 1955, 2006; Längle & Sykes, 2006). He recalled one particularly grueling day of work when the idea that love can contribute to meaning was illuminated:

> We were at work in a trench. The dawn was grey around us; grey was the sky above; grey the snow in the pale light of dawn; grey the rags in which my fellow prisoners were clad, and grey their faces. I was again conversing silently with my wife, or perhaps I was struggling to find the *reason* for my sufferings, my slow dying. In a last violent protest against the hopelessness of imminent death, I sensed my spirit piercing through the enveloping gloom. I felt it transcend that hopeless, meaningless world, and from somewhere I heard a victorious "Yes" in answer to my question of the existence of an ultimate purpose (2006, p. 40).

Reflections on the dehumanizing conditions of Auschwitz led Frankl to the conviction that there must be a meaning in suffering (Frankl, 1959, 1973, 2006). He recalled instances where life and death seemed interchangeable, such as seeing a corpse and then realizing he had conversed with the dead man just two hours earlier. He wrote about the insecure existence inmates experienced, reduced to the numbers tattooed on their arms. Frankl explained the paradoxical insignificance and significance of those numbers: "One literally became a number: dead or alive, that was unimportant; the life of 'a number' was completely irrelevant. What stood behind that number and that life mattered even less: the fate, the history, the name of the man" (2006, p. 53).

Frankl's logotherapy was greatly influenced by the existential philosopher Nietzsche. He found that Nietzsche's tenet, "He who has a why to live for can bear with almost any how" (2006, p.76), was especially pertinent in a concentration camp. Frankl recalled a fellow inmate who had observed so many deaths that he could decipher the differences and similarities in each person's relationship to life. Thus, this inmate knew that when a prisoner had given up hope, death was imminent. This observation on the necessity of hope supported Frankl's philosophy of meaning.

THE TRIDIMENSIONAL ONTOLOGY OF LOGOTHERAPY

Frankl (1946/1973) conceived of a paradigm to better understand the uniquely human aspects of individuals that logotherapy targets. The tridimensional ontology of logotherapy views individuals as being comprised of three separate but interacting realms: *biological/physical, psychological,* and *spiritual.* The biological and psychological dimensions are evident in all mammals: a living being has both a physical presence and cognitive psychological abilities. This is true of all animals and beasts. However, what separates humans from other living beings is the third dimension: an individual's essence lies within the *spiritual* dimension, which Frankl (1946/1973) believed was "specifically human" (p. xi). This dimension encompasses the unique characteristics of an individual, including values, passions and—most importantly to psychotherapy—meaning. In his holistic approach, Frankl ensured that each dimension of his patients' existence was recognized. As a physician, he was able to address the physical and psychological deficiencies in his patients. As a logotherapist, he addressed struggles within the spiritual dimension.

Alex Vesely Frankl explained to me that his grandfather did not intend to equate the term *spirituality* with *religion*. The German words *geistig* and *geistlich* both translate to *spiritual* in English; however, *gesistlich* has religious connotations. Frankl therefore preferred *geistig*, to avoid an association with religion. The English language does not utilize two distinct words for *spirituality* and therefore the term is often assumed to relate to religion. To avoid this implication, English-speaking logotherapists often substitute the word *noetic*, which refers to *noology*, or the study of the mind and intellect (Zaiser, 2005). Therefore, Frankl's tridimensional ontology can be described as being made up of the physical dimension, the psychological dimension and the spiritual or noetic dimension.

Fabry, a close associate of Frankl, articulated that the spiritual, noetic dimension houses the following qualities:

> ... our will to meaning, our goal orientation, ideas and ideals, creativity, imagination, faith, love that goes beyond the physical, a conscience beyond the superego, self-transcendence, commitments, responsibility, a sense of humor, and the freedom of choice making (1987, p. 19)

Uncovering the contents of the spiritual dimension allows us to better understand its function and distinguish it from the physical and psychological dimensions of humanity. In reading Fabry's words, I discerned a correlation between the qualities of the spiritual dimension and my examination of Holocaust artwork. Creativity and imagination are inherent in art, indicating that any art-making process is a function of the spiritual dimension. Beyond that, I noticed other qualities which Fabry identified in my categorization of Holocaust art in Chapter 3, the examples of communal art making in Chapter 4 and the findings of my phenomenological study as detailed in Chapter 7. Love can be seen in the examples of portraiture, as well as in the cultural communities that developed in camps and ghettos. Satirical works, like those of Paval Fantl, indicate a sense of humor; while the need to document suggests a responsibility and conscience. The freedom of choice can be seen in the works of all the artists who chose to create, as they exercised the few freedoms they had to make art.

Frankl's tridimensional ontology and the significance of the spiritual or noetic dimension are exemplified through the phenomenon of Holocaust art. The individuals creating artwork in camps and ghettos were starved, abused and humiliated, and yet still found personal meaning within their suffering. Camp and ghetto inmates were typically in poor physical health due to malnutrition, inadequate hygiene, exhausting manual labor and frequent beatings. The torture also affected their psychological health, as they contended with the constant threat of danger. The lingering impact of loss and destruction of their former lives also harmed their psyche. Looking at the physical and psychological dimensions of camp and ghetto residents, one could assert that these victims were quite ill. However, logotherapy contends that, unlike our physical and psychological dimensions, the noetic dimension of an individual can never become sick. In the pursuit of meaning, "the defiant power of the human spirit is evoked to rebel against seemingly all powerful forces of the psyche and body" (Fabry, 1987, p. 26). By engaging in art practices, these artists activated the distinctly human aspect of themselves to find meaning in their circumstances. Though their motivation differed, each artist engaged in creativity as a means of enduring. The sense of meaning that these artists found stemmed from the spiritual dimension, which has the capacity to prevail despite physical and psychological limitations (Fabry, 1987; Frankl, 1973).

MEANING

According to Frankl (1959/2006), survival in an extreme environment is possible only if an individual can find meaning. Meaning can offer stability and grounding in a chaotic world (Hoffman, Stewart, Warren & Meek, 2009), and is therefore "the ultimate coping mechanism" (p. 260). This stance is echoed in the art therapy literature (Appleton, 2001; Kalmanowitz & Ho, 2016; Moon, 2009; Wilkinson & Chilton, 2013, 2018). Appleton (2001) observed that an art therapy group supported adolescents in identifying a personal meaning in response to a traumatic event. Wilkinson and Chilton (2013) asserted that creativity can "illuminate purpose and meaning" (p. 5), leading to an improved quality of life.

The term *meaning* is both obvious and vague. In my experience, it is a concept that is understood as important, but is rarely explicitly defined. This may in part be because meaning is highly personal and varies based on the individual: what one person identifies as meaningful may be meaningless to another. The subjective and personal nature of meaning makes it critical to an existentially oriented psychotherapy. Yalom and Josselson noted that individuals frequently seek psychotherapy in an attempt to address issues that relate to a lack of meaning and purpose (2004). Therefore, the search for meaning can be an integral part of the therapeutic process.

The term *meaning making* is frequently used to describe activities, experiences and sensations that evoke meaning. However, logotherapy is built on the concept of *meaning finding*, rather than *meaning making*. This seemingly subtle difference is significant in how one understands personal meaning. Frankl insisted that meaning cannot be made, because it already exists. Humans are unique in that we are capable of finding meaning in even the most challenging circumstances. Therefore, the search for meaning is the task of logotherapy. Frankl believed that it is the logotherapist's responsibility to guide clients through this search to find meaning.

For Frankl, meaning is simply *what is meant*. This can be what is meant in a specific moment or what is meant of one's life. Fabry (1987) distinguished *meaning of the moment* and *ultimate meaning*. *Meaning of the moment* pertains to the choices one makes in mundane, day-to-day situations. In every moment, one has the opportunity to make a meaningful choice. *Ultimate meaning* relates to one's role and purpose within the ecosystem of their world. Finding ultimate meaning is a life task which requires "a constant search in which it does make a difference what we decide to do and refuse to do" (Fabry, 1987, p. 35). Ultimate meaning comprises the millions of choices one makes throughout their life.

Yalom's definition of *meaning* is aligned with the logotherapeutic view. Meaning involves committing to a cause; having a set goal or purpose; and fighting for something outside of oneself (Yalom & Josselson, 2004). Meaning can be found only when one looks beyond their own needs to their larger world. Frankl and subsequent logotherapists believed that meaning is the force that motivates human behavior and action (Wong, 2012, 2014). This contradicts the Freudian notion that behavior is driven by pleasure or the Adlerian notion that power is a driving force. Frankl believed that the goal of life is to find a meaning that makes life worth living.

Happiness, he argued, is a side effect of finding meaning. To focus exclusively on one's happiness suggests a selfishness that disregards the importance of connection in finding meaning.

Batthyany and Russo-Netzer (2014) define *meaning* as "a metaphorical lighthouse that sheds light on life events and enables people to draw strengths and insights from their positive and negative experiences, gain perspective from present situations, and point to a worthwhile and valuable future" (p. 9.) This definition highlights the personalized nature of meaning, in that it stems from an individual's life experience. I ultimately define *meaning* as an internal construct that brings cohesion to life experiences. Meaning, or the search for meaning, drives decision making, shapes personal values and grounds an individual to a place of authenticity. Meaning is found in passions, ideals, values, memories and relationships. Meaning is found when an act, a relationship or an interaction feels like what is meant.

The element of choice is critical to meaningfulness. By experiencing freedom of choice, humans are given regular opportunities to respond to adverse situations in ways that align with personal values, thereby achieving meaning (Schulenberg et al, 2008). However, when a person's responses conflict with their individual values, goals and overall essence, the result is a sense of meaninglessness. According to Frankl, psychiatric conditions grow out of the antithesis of meaning: *meaninglessness*. Meaninglessness is found in the absence of purpose, cohesion and explanation (Berry-Smith, 2012), and can result in feelings of dysphoria, helplessness and spiritual emptiness. Frankl (1972) identified two stages of existential meaninglessness as they appear in psychotherapy. An *existential vacuum* (Frankl, 1973; Yalom, 1980) is a state of apathy and hopelessness in which one experiences no sense of intent or purpose. In an attempt to fill the existential vacuum, an individual enters *existential neurosis*, which is characterized by depression, angst and/or maladaptive behavior. In this construct, Frankl viewed psychiatric symptoms as a reaction to the experience of meaninglessness. Thus, he emphasized that humans must identify a personal meaning for existence and live accordingly. Without a perception of meaning, a person lacks substance and subsequently loses motivation and drive to live an authentic existence.

The artists of the Holocaust found meaning by stepping outside themselves, or *self-transcending*, to commit to a larger goal. The meaning they identified gave them a reason to fight for their survival. The *muselmann*, however, succumbed to a state of meaninglessness and lost their will to survive. Through the example of art making in the Holocaust, we can understand the importance of finding meaning in order to withstand suffering.

MEANING IN POSITIVE PSYCHOLOGY

While my conception of meaning making is informed by existential and logotherapeutic theory, it is important to note that other areas of psychology also utilize the construct of meaning. The field of positive psychology has embraced the concept of meaning, finding it paramount to a happy life (Wilkinson & Chilton, 2018). Martela & Steger (2016) developed their own trichotomy in which they base meaning on three facets: *coherence, purpose* and *significance*. Though this construct is geared toward positive psychology, it is built on existential theories. *Coherence* refers to a degree of predictability in one's life. An individual can find meaning when patterns are recognized and lead to a feeling of wholeness that allows them to make sense of their life (Martela & Steger, 2016; Heintzelman & King, 2014).

The second facet, *purpose*, stems from Frankl's articulation that meaning arises when one can identify a clear purpose in their life (2006). Though *purpose* and *meaning* are often used interchangeably (Reker & Peacock, 1981), in this framework, purpose drives meaning. *Purpose* is an internal force that organizes and rouses ambitions, motivates actions and ultimately gives an individual a sense of meaning (Mcknight & Kashdan, 2009).

The third facet to meaning, *significance*, relates to the "value, worth, and importance" of one's life (Martela & Steger, 2016, p. 535). Life is worth living when it is value laden and worthwhile. *Significance* is akin to the idea of *existential mattering*, which considers the value of one's existence (George & Park, 2014).

Martela and Steger's theory on the facets of meaning overlaps with tenets of logotherapy, highlighting an integration of positive psychology with existentialism (e.g., Batthyany & Russo-Netzer, 2014; Wong, 2014, 2012, 2009). Wong's (2012) dual systems approach aims to link the meaning-making emphasis of logotherapy with the pillars of positive psychology. Since, as Frankl asserted, meaning making is a distinctly human ability, it is appropriate for inclusion as a factor in all humanistic branches of psychology. Wong (2104) noted that as the idea of meaning making becomes increasingly popular in psychology research, it can only be advanced through a deeper understanding of Frankl's construct of, and the search for, meaning.

CONCLUSIONS

It is clear that Viktor Frankl's work challenged existing psychological theories and brought the concept of meaning to the forefront. His impact on the different fields of psychology is evident in existential theory, positive psychology and, of course, logotherapy. His theories have also provided a framework to support my understanding of Holocaust artwork. Inversely, the phenomenon of Holocaust artwork serves to explicate theories of logotherapy. This chapter has served to acquaint the reader with existential theory and logotherapy, and to link those theories to the art of the Holocaust. Existential theory and logotherapy both avoid manualized approaches in favor of one tailored to the individual client. As Schneider & Krug (2017) asserted, the existential therapist should rely on engagement with the client to guide their practice. Frankl was known to be a keen observer and argued that if two individuals in therapy were being treated the same way, at least one of them was being treated wrongly. He built his theory on his observation of humans in a range of conditions. I have aimed to develop my own art therapy theories based on my research into the phenomenon of art making within the Holocaust. My goal was to understand this phenomenon to inform my own theories and practice. In doing so, I found meaning in my research—a process that was congruent with existential and logotherapy philosophy. I have since relied on my research, as well as those two strands of theory, to guide my clinical work. In the following chapters, I will describe how logotherapy and the search for meaning can be incorporated into art therapy practices.

REFERENCES

Appleton, V. (2001) Avenues of hope: Art therapy and the resolution of trauma, *Art Therapy*, *18*(1), 6–13, doi: 10.1080/07421656.2001.10129454

Amishai-Maisels, Z. (1993). *Depiction and interpretation: The influence of the Holocaust on visual arts.* Tarrytown, NY: Pergamon Press.

Batthyany, A. & Russo-Netzer, P. (eds.). (2014). *Meaning in positive and existential psychology.* New York, NY: Springer.

Berry-Smith, S. F. (2012). *Death, freedom, isolation and meaninglessness and the existential psychotherapy of Irvin D. Yalom* (Doctoral dissertation, Auckland University of Technology).

Cooper, M. (2015). *Existential psychotherapy and counselling: Contributions to a pluralistic practice.* London, England: Sage.

Dalek, J. & Swiebocka, T. (1989) *Suffering and hope: Artistic creations of the Oświęcim prisoners.* (Jolanta Kosiec, trans.). Oświęcim, Poland: Panstwowe Muzeum Auschwitz-Birkenau.

Dissanayake, E. (1995). *Homo aestheticus: Where art comes from and why.* Seattle, WA: University of Washington Press.

Fabry, J. B. (1987). *The Pursuit of meaning: Viktor Frank, logotherapy, and life.* Berkeley, CA: Institute of Logotherapy Press.

Frankl, V. (1973). *The doctor and the soul. From psychotherapy to logotherapy.* New York, NY: Vintage Books.

Frankl, V. (1959/2006). *Man's search for meaning* (5th ed.) (I. Lasch, trans.). Boston, MA: Beacon Press.

Frankl, V. E. (1966). Self-transcendence as a human phenomenon. *Journal of Humanistic Psychology*, *6*(2), 97–106.

Frankl, V. (1967). *Psychotherapy and existentialism: Selected papers on logotherapy.* New York, NY: Simon and Schuster.

Frankl, V. E. (1988). The will to meaning: Foundations and applications of logotherapy. New York, NY: Meridian

Frankl, V. (2004). *On the theory and therapy of mental disorders: An introduction to logotherapy and existential analysis.* (J. Dubois, trans.). New York, NY: Routledge.

Frankl, V. E. (2014). *The will to meaning: Foundations and applications of logotherapy.* London, England: Penguin.

George, L. S. & Park, C. L. (2014). Existential mattering: Bringing attention to a neglected but central aspect of meaning? In A. Batthyany & P. Russo-Netzer (eds.). *Meaning in positive and existential psychology.* New York, NY: Springer, pp. 39–51.

Grant, M. (2002). *I knew I was painting for my life: The Holocaust artworks of Marianne Grant.* Glasgow, Scotland: Glasgow Museums.

Hanson, B. (2006). Dissonance and aesthetic totality: Adorno reads Schonberg. In J. Hermand & G. Richter (eds.). *Sound figures of modernity: German music and philosophy.* Madison, WI: Univeristy of Wisconsin Press.

Heintzelman, S. J. & King, L. A. (2014). (The feeling of) Meaning-as-information. *Personality and Social Psychology Review*, *18*, 153–167.

Hoffman, L., Stewart, S., Warren, D. & Meek, L. (2009). Toward a sustainable myth of self: An existential response to the postmodern condition. *Journal of Humanistic Psychology*, *49*(2), 135–173. doi: 10.1177/0022167808324880

Jones, A. (2001). Absurdity and being-in-itself. The third phase of phenomenology: Jean-Paul Sartre and existential psychoanalysis. *Journal of Psychiatric & Mental Health Nursing*, *8*(4), 367–372. doi: 10.1046/j.1365-2850.2001.00405.x

Kalmanowitz, D. & Ho, R. T. (2016). Out of our mind. Art therapy and mindfulness with refugees, political violence and trauma. *The Arts in Psychotherapy*, *49*, 57–65. doi: 10.1016/j. aip.2016.05.012

Längle, A. & Sykes, B. M. (2006). Viktor Frankl—advocate for humanity: On his 100th birthday. *Journal of Humanistic Psychology*, *46*(1), 36–47.

Levi, P. (1985). *Moments of reprieve*. New York, NY: Penguin Books.

Martela, F. & Steger, M. F. (2016). The three meanings of meaning in life: Distinguishing coherence, purpose, and significance. *The Journal of Positive Psychology*, *11*(5), 531–545, doi: 10.1080/17439760.2015.1137623

May, R. & Yalom, I. (2000). Existential psychotherapy. In R. J. Corsini & D. Wedding (eds.). *Current psychotherapies* (6th ed., pp. 279–302). Itasca, Ill: Peacock.

Mcknight, P. E. & Kashdan, T. B. (2009). Purpose in life as a system that creates and sustains health and well-being: An integrative, testable theory. *Review of General Psychology*, *13*, 242–251.

Moon, B. (2009). *Existential art therapy: The canvas mirror*. Springfield, IL: Charles C. Thomas.

Novitch, M., Dawidowicz, L. S. & Freudenheim, T. L. (1981). *Spiritual resistance: Art from concentration camps, 1940–1945: A selection of drawings and paintings from the collection of Kibbutz Lohamei Haghetaot, Israel*. Philadelphia, PA: Jewish Publication Society.

Reker, G. T. & Peacock, E. J. (1981). The life attitude profile (LAP): A multidimensional instrument for assessing attitudes toward life. *Canadian Journal of Behavioural Science/Revue Canadienne Des Sciences Du Comportement*, *13*, 264–273. doi: 10.1037/h0081178

Sartre, J. P. (1949). *Literature and existentialism*. New York, NY: Citadel Press.

Seligman, Z. (1995). Trauma and drama: A lesson from the concentration camps. *The Arts in psychotherapy*, *22*(2), 119–132. doi: 10.1016/0197-4556(95)00017-Y

Schneider, K. J. & Krug, O. T. (2017). *Existential-humanistic therapy*. Washington, DC: American Psychological Association.

Schneider, K. (2015). The case for existential (spiritual) psychotherapy. *Journal of Contemporary Psychotherapy*, *45*(1), 21–24. doi: 10.1007/s10879-014-9278-8

Smith, M. J. (1972). *The harrowing of hell: Dachau*. Albuquerque, NM: University of New Mexico Press.

Sousa, D. (2015). Existential psychotherapy the genetic-phenomenological approach: Beyond a dichotomy between relating and skills. *Journal of Contemporary Psychotherapy 45*(1), 69–77. doi: 10.1007/s10879-014-9283-y

Van Deurzen, E. (2007). Existential therapy. In W. Dryden (ed.). *Dryden's handbook of individual therapy* (195–225). London, England: Sage.

van Deurzen, E. (2012). *Existential counselling & psychotherapy in practice* (3rd ed.). London, England: Sage.

van Deurzen, E. & Arnold-Baker, C. (2018). *Existential therapy: Distinctive features*. New York, NY: Routledge.

Wilkinson, R. A. & Chilton, G. (2013). Positive art therapy: Linking positive psychology to art therapy theory, practice, and research. *Art Therapy*, *30*(1), 4–11.

Wilkinson, R. A. & Chilton, G. (2018). *Positive art therapy theory and practice: Integrating positive psychology with art therapy*. New York, NY: Routledge.

Wong, P. T. (2009). Meaning therapy: An integrative and positive existential psychotherapy. *Journal of Contemporary Psychotherapy*, *40*(2), 85–93. doi: 10.1007/s10879-009-9132-6

Wong, P. T. (2012). Toward a dual-systems model of what makes life worth living. In *The human quest for meaning* (pp. 49–68). New York, NY: Routledge.

Wong, P. T. P. (2014). Viktor Frankl's meaning seeking model and positive psychology. In A. Batthyany & P. Russo Netzer (eds.). *Meaning in existential and positive psychology*. New York, NY: Springer.

Yalom, I. (1980). *Existential psychotherapy*. New York, NY: Basic Books.

Yalom, I. D. (2008). Staring at the sun: Overcoming the terror of death. *The Humanistic Psychologist, 36*(3–4), 283–297.

Yalom, I. & Josselson, R. (2013). Existential psychotherapy. In D. Wedding & R. J. Corsini (eds.). *Current Psychotherapies, 10ᵗʰ edition*. Belmont, CA: Brooks/Cole.

Zaiser, R. (2005). Working on the noetic dimension of man: Philosophical practice, logotherapy, and existential analysis. *Philosophical practice, 1*(2), 83–88.

CHAPTER 9

INTEGRATING LOGOTHERAPY AND ART THERAPY

In the previous chapter, I described the emergence of the logotherapy philosophy developed by Holocaust survivor and acclaimed psychiatrist Viktor Frankl. To review, logotherapy—which loosely translates as *meaning therapy*—grew out of existential theory and emphasizes the individual's search for meaning. Logotherapy has since been developed beyond Frankl's initial conception in 1926 and is used in contemporary practices in conjunction with existential theory; positive psychology (Wong, 2009, 2014); acceptance commitment therapy (Sharp, Wilson & Schulenberg, 2004); and cognitive behavior therapy (Ameli, 2016). Remarkably, logotherapy is not featured in art therapy literature, despite the commonality of finding meaning through creativity. Frankl specifically asserted that meaning can be achieved through creativity, experience and attitude (1973). Meaning in logotherapy has a direct correlation to health and wellbeing (Pfeifer, 2021). Meaning is known to promote resilience and can function as a preventative measure to psychiatric health concerns (Thir & Batthyany, 2016). Melton and Schulenberg (2008) found that meaning is associated with a stable mood, reduced psychological distress, improved social behaviors and a more proactive attitude. As art therapists guide their clients through the creative process to communicate their experiences and express themselves in an attempt to find meaning, they are unknowingly working within a logotherapeutic framework.

My desire to formally incorporate logotherapy philosophy into art therapy discourse came as a result of my research on the phenomenon of art making within the Holocaust. Through my phenomenological study, I came across extensive examples of individuals finding meaning in their circumstances through art making. The narratives I was told or read about all contained elements that logotherapists attribute to meaning. Art making to find meaning was also discussed in the literature on Holocaust art (Moreh Rosenberg, 2016; Amishai-Maisels, 1993). Additionally, themes of meaning surfaced in conversations and informal interviews with Holocaust art scholars and curators at Yad Vashem, Beit Terezín and the United States Holocaust Museum and Memorial. My findings were consistent in that creating artwork in a camp or ghetto led the artist to find meaning. Once found, that sense of meaning contributed to psychic survival.

PSYCHIC SURVIVAL

Framing the act of creating art within the Holocaust as an attempt to find meaning helps us to understand the motivation of the Holocaust artists. From a pragmatic standpoint, it is baffling that artists would take the time—and the risk—to create. Frankl (1973) explained that in a concentration or extermination camp, one's every move was geared toward survival. There was no room for trivial, unrelated ideas in the prisoners' minds, so all thoughts and instincts were intrinsically related to surviving the day. If the actions of camp inmates were fueled primarily by a survival need, then where did art making fit in? If we are to believe that every conscious act was

DOI: 10.4324/9781003160885-13

geared toward survival, then did making art contribute to survival? Was the act of creating artwork also an act of survival? Perhaps not directly; but through the lens of logotherapy, it is fair to say that art making contributed to psychic survival—which, according to Frankl, was a critical component of survival in the camp systems (2006). Kosiec alluded to art making leading to spiritual survival when, in reference to the Auschwitz art collection, he pondered: "Perhaps the instinct for life is something more than simply the struggle for biological survival?" (1989, p. 1).

Examples of art making leading to spiritual survival within the Holocaust are numerous. Cellist Herman Boesson was recruited to play in the Auschwitz orchestra, which played patriotic marches during roll calls—a particularly tortuous time for prisoners. Boesson stated that the ability to play music during his captivity "saved my life in the camps, both physically as well as spiritually" (as cited in Costanza, 1982, p. 13). Physically, Boesson's skill rendered him useful to his captors and therefore his life was spared. Spiritually, he was saved by being able to offer his unique skill to those around him, including fellow prisoners. An artist in Auschwitz, Mieczysław Kościel-niak, referred to the spiritual power art making offered, stating in a testimony: "Just like for me and many other inmates, the very opportunity of following creative pursuits gave spiritual power, and hence it was essential to the struggle to survive and retain dignity" (as cited in Sieradzka, 2019). Another example is the case of Alfred Kantor, who described how drawing in Auschwitz supported his psyche: "By taking on the role of 'observer', I could at least for a few moments detach myself from what was going on in Auschwitz and was therefore better able to hold together the threads of sanity" (1971, para 31). Transcending his circumstances by imagining himself as observer, rather than victim, Kantor found a meaning in his suffering, which allowed for psychic survival.

These examples of spiritual power support Frankl's notion of psychic survival. Frankl did not explicitly define *psychic survival* in his writings, though my conversation with Alex Vesely Frankl helped me to better conceptualize the term. Frankl was adamant that finding meaning in life can make any situation bearable and therefore life worth living. When one finds meaning, they have a reason to live. Within the Holocaust, those who could not identify a meaning had no motivation to push themselves toward survival. Meaning is subjective, so each individual's motivation to survive differed. While this text focuses on meaning through art making, there are extensive examples of Holocaust victims finding meaning in myriad ways: through performance art; a commitment to saving the Jewish race; a hope to create a Zionist state; or the determination to reunite with loved ones. The commonality in these examples is that, once found, each individual's meaning led them to want to survive. Therefore, *psychic survival* refers to the desire to survive regardless of the degree of suffering that ensues. Frankl used the equation *despair = suffering − meaning*. Suffering is inevitable, but despair is avoidable. Meaning enables individuals to endure suffering.

Although Frankl's use of the phrase *psychic survival* was specific to Holocaust victims, it underscores the existential and logotherapeutic emphasis on meaning being centric to life. My study of Holocaust art has indicated that art making is a way to find meaning, which thus contributes to psychic survival. With this idea in mind, I would like to return to the discussion of art as a functional behavior that I referenced in Chapter 1. Dissanayake (1995) posited that art making has an evolutionary function and pointedly defined art making as a behavior. She stated that categorizing art as a behavior suggests that artistically prone humans survive better than others: "in the evolution of the human species, art-inclined individuals, those who possessed this behavior of art, survived better than those who did not" (1995, p. 35). When art is classified as a human behavior, we recognize it as intrinsically important to human existence. In this argument, Dissanayake suggested that the behavior of art making is somehow linked to biological survival, as art making has historically been a consistent human behavior. In a similar vein, Kaimal (2019) noted that creativity is engrained in the human brain and proposed that art making be viewed as an adaptive response to threatening situations. Both arguments support the act of art making and creativity as survival trait.

Linking these arguments to logotherapy philosophy, we can postulate how art making contributes to human survival. In the case of the Holocaust, art making led individuals to find meaning, thus giving them a motivation to survive. Perhaps Dissanayake noticed a connection between art making and survival because those who find meaning in art have a reason to survive.

Frankl's specific notion of meaning as a motivating factor in survival suggests that art making has evolved into a biological necessity (Dissanayake, 1995), because it allows individuals to find meaning. This framework supports an integration of logotherapy into art therapy practices. There are additional areas in which logotherapy philosophy aligns with art therapy theory. In the following sections, I will identify other aspects of logotherapy that relate to art therapy, beginning with how art making has been incorporated into logotherapeutic practices.

ART IN LOGOTHERAPY

Frankl was known to hold an appreciation for the arts, viewing such pursuits as expressions of humanity. In fact, I discovered in my conversation with his grandson that Frankl and I share the same favorite artist, Austrian figure painter Egon Schiele. Frankl believed that viewing or making art could help individuals to rediscover their own sense of humanity (Frankl, 2006; Pfeifer, 2021). To reinforce these ideas, he integrated creative practices within his therapeutic approach. The Mountain Range Exercise was first introduced in his book *The Doctor and the Soul* (1973) and was later developed as an activity by Ernzen (1990). In this exercise, a client is asked to draw a mountain range and then to draw or write the names of people they deem important on the peaks. These people can be family members, friends or public figures—anyone whom the client holds in high regard. After the names are written on the mountain drawing, the therapist engages the client in a discussion of why these people are important, asking questions such as, "What values does this person embody?" or "What do you have in common with this person?" The goal of this activity is to help the individual clarify their own values and consider the positive relationships in their life. The Mountain Range Exercise has been used on inpatient units and in substance abuse treatment (Ernzen, 1990), as well as with sex offenders (Schulenberg, 2003, 2004).

I have used the Mountain Range Exercise in art therapy sessions to help clients identify meaningful relationships in their lives, as well as attributes they admire in those people. Within the given directive, I allow my clients freedom of choice in materials and the resulting images are always unique. Some clients choose to use different media for the mountains and people, while others prefer a uniform approach. Some clients incorporate themselves into the mountain range, indicating an appreciation for the self and the relationships that they are part of. I worked with one client who struggled to identify admirable people she knew in her life, but was able to use magazine photos of celebrities to represent the qualities they embodied or to stand in for relationships she hoped to form. The informal structure of this exercise makes its accessible and typically leads to a discussion about connections, relationships and values.

Another art directive used in logotherapy is the Family Shoebox Game. Developed by Lanz (1993), the Family Shoebox Game incorporates logotherapy into a family therapy session. In this activity, a family is given a shoebox along with scissors, glue, and magazines. The therapist instructs the family to work together to glue images depicting their family values inside the shoebox and glue images of external values on the outside of the shoebox. This was seen as a way to observe how the family interacts and to facilitate a conversation about family values and meaning (Lantz, 1993; Schuelnberg et al, 2016). I do not typically facilitate family therapy sessions, so I have not tried this in my practice.

Artistic process and creativity are connected to meaning in existential literature beyond Frankl. May (1974) theorized that there is a highly relevant relationship between creativity and existentialism. In his view, the creative process is paramount to finding meaning. Like Frankl, May asserted that life struggles can ultimately foster meaning, and that meaning can be found through creativity. The capacity to recognize beauty results in meaning, regardless of the despair that may have bred it. May described authentic creativity as "bringing something new into being" (1974, p. 38) and argued that creativity represents a high level of emotional health and self-actualization. May also pondered the place of death anxiety in creativity, asserting that the purpose of creativity is "the passion to live beyond one's death" (1974, p. 31). He believed that creative engagement offers a sense of wholeness. It evokes a sensation of ecstasy and joy (May, 1974), and results in a grounding, comprehensive understanding of the self. Contemporary existentialists Schneider and Krug argue that a main assumption in existential therapy is that "human beings have the potential to grow and re-create themselves through ongoing creative practices" (2017, p. 25). Art therapy—an inherently creative practice—can therefore support this process of growth in one's search for meaning.

While art making has been part of the logotherapy process, logotherapy is rarely referred to by name in art therapy literature. Still, the core tenants of logotherapy are congruous with those of art therapy principles. Art therapists subscribe to the importance of finding meaning in their practice (Betensky, 2001; Fenner, 2012; Moon, 2009; Wilkinson & Chilton, 2013). Betensky (2001) described watching the recognition of meaning in her clients as they reflected on their artwork in an art therapy session: "I also find that the emergence of meanings, even small ones, as when a line or a color suddenly becomes visible, enables clients to see unrealized possibilities or untapped potencies" (2001, pp. 123-124). In this description, Betensky articulated how art making can help clients recognize their potential for change—which, as Schulenberg et al. (2016) point out, is the responsibility of the logotherapist.

In addition to the emphasis on meaning, there are other aspects of logotherapy which complement art therapy. Themes essential to logotherapy—such as self-transcendence, authenticity and freedom—are innate to the art-making process.

Additionally, Frankl's tridimensional ontology of logotherapy, which I described in the previous chapter, is mirrored in the American Art Therapy Association's description of art therapy as an engagement "of the mind, body, and spirit in ways that are distinct from verbal articulation alone" (2018). This language is similar to Frankl's designation of the three elements of humanity as physical, psychological and spiritual. Perhaps our practice is more related to logotherapy than we realized.

VALUES TOWARD FINDING MEANING

The will toward meaning is a crucial element in logotherapy. One must have a desire, or will, to find meaning and recognize one's own capacity to do so. In logotherapy, meaning is not made, but rather found. Frankl (1988) articulated that meaning can be found through one of three different values: *creative, experiential* and *attitudinal*. Frankl explained:

> If one prefers in this context to speak of values, he may discern three chief groups of values. I have classified them in terms of creative, experiential, and attitudinal values. This sequence reflects the three principal ways in which man can find meaning in life. The first is what he gives to the world in terms of his creations; the second is what he takes from the world in terms of encounters and experiences; and the third is the stand he takes to his predicament in case he must face a fate which he cannot change (1988, p. 70).

Purjo (2013) noted that the word *values* in this context may be misleading. Given that Frankl's works were translated from his native German, we once again notice word choices that can be misinterpreted when read in English. In this particular instance, the creative, experiential and attitudinal *values* that Frankl described are more accurately *principles* that can lead to a values-based meaning in life (Purjo, 2013). Purjo elaborated that one's true sense of meaning and purpose in life is achieved through doing something valuable and therefore meaningful for oneself and the common good. The creative, experiential and attitudinal values, or principles, each represent a pathway through which an individual can find and access meaning (DuBoise, 2004).

I have made the argument that Holocaust artists found meaning in their existence by making art. Frankl's aforementioned values toward finding meaning further explicate how these artists were able to do so. Giving to the world creatively, encountering the people and experiences around them, and taking a stand in response to their unforgiving circumstances were the pathways in which these artists were able to find meaning. The artists creating in the Holocaust can exemplify how these values were activated in the pursuit of meaning.

Creativity

The creative value is realized by bringing something new into existence and thereby making a contribution to the world (Frankl, 1973, 1988). Although the word *creativity* leads us to think of the arts, this value refers to the broader act of creating and bringing something new into existence (Dubois, 2004). The creative value is evident in art making, as well as construction, gardening and even parenting. The sole principle is that meaning can be found by creating something new and giving it a place in the world. As the focus of this text is on art and art therapy, my elaboration will remain on the concept of creativity via art making; though it is important to note that artistic pursuits are not the only way in which an individual can find meaning through creation.

The value of creativity is the most obvious way in which Holocaust artists found meaning. Though their supplies—and often their time—were limited, artists in camps and ghettos fully engaged in creative pursuits by drawing, painting and sculpting. Lamberti (1995) argued that the benefits of making art in camps and ghettos were realized through the process of creating. The simple act of creating, regardless of the scope or size of the creation itself, led Holocaust artists to find meaning. The term *creative impulse* arose in my conversation with Samuel Bak, which he described as "a need to communicate, even to communicate with oneself" (S. Bak, personal communication, October 10, 2017). Indeed, through their work, these artists communicated with each other, and with future viewers. I have previously mentioned the odd juxtaposition of creation in an environment designed for destruction. For some artists, I believe that creating anything at all showed their commitment to opposing destruction. That commitment, and the act of creating artwork to honor it, allowed artists to find meaning. There is no doubt that the artwork created by these artists was an act of creativity, passion and commitment.

Of note, Tomic (2019) found that creative engagement in camps and ghettos not only led to a psychic survival, but also supported psychological wellbeing after liberation, noting that those who made art during captivity—and continued to do so after liberation—were able to adjust better to their new life. This has two implications. First, finding meaning not only supported survival within the Holocaust, but also supported individuals who survived the Holocaust in their transition to post-war life. Second, the fact that meaning was found through art making both in captivity and beyond highlights the authenticity of that meaning. Finding meaning through art making was, as Frankl would say, meant to be.

Some artists also found additional meaning through their artwork after liberation, as they were able to use their work to implicate their captors. Yehuda Bacon's detailed drawings of the gas chambers and crematoria at Auschwitz were used as evidence in the Eichmann trials; as were Esther Lurie's watercolors (USHMM, n.d.). Mira Jovanović's drawings from the Banjica camp were submitted as material evidence against the camp commander (Tomić, et al, 2019). It was not uncommon for Holocaust survivors to question why they survived when so many others had perished (Juni, 2016; Kellermann 2001). Using their artwork to communicate the atrocities they endured allowed them to find meaning in survival.

Experiential

According to Frankl, experiential values "are realized by the passive receiving of the world (nature, art) into the ego" (p. 105). In this pathway, meaning is found through our awareness of our world experiences and sensations (Frankl, 1973; Pfeifer, 2021). Pfeifer (2021) described the experiential values as comprising *receptivity*, *contemplation*, and *emotionality*. By experiencing our world, we receive it, contemplate it and develop an emotional attachment to it. Examples of this value include the immersive process of viewing art or listening to music; the connectedness one gets from appreciating nature; and the feeling of connecting deeply and mutually with another person.

Frankl's examples of the experiential value included the way humans experience art, nature and interpersonal relationships. The experiential component of art making—from the impression of a pencil in one's hand to the ability to take in the artwork made—is one way in which Holocaust artists found meaning in art making. The subtle sensations inherent in art making allowed artists to fully immerse themselves in their work. The scent of the art materials may have evoked memories of a classroom or studio. The feel of an instrument in one's hand may have been a reminder of a favorite pencil or paintbrush. The opportunity to reflect on their art, and share it, supported a connectedness to oneself and to others. This may have been especially true for professional artists, such as Otto Ungar, Bedrich Fritta, Friedl Dicker-Brandeis and Xawery Dunikowski, among others. Engagement in art making connected them to the meaningful life they lived as artists prior to their captivity. The sensory aspects of the art process likely contrasted against the harshness and austerity of their environments, and reignited a passion in them that helped them find meaning within their circumstances.

The numerous portraits created in the Holocaust highlight the human connection that is part of the experiential value. By creating portraits of fellow inmates, artists allowed themselves to fully experience another individual. The act of sitting with another to witness and acknowledge their suffering led to a sense of receptivity, as a new relationship was formed between artist and subject. Leclerc (2011) noted that portraits allowed both artist and sitter to witness each other's experience, which can be viewed as a form of receptivity. In this example, I am also reminded of Halina Olomucki, who was asked by fellow female prisoners at Birkenau to draw their portraits in an attempt to affirm and, on her part, acknowledge their existence (Figure 9.1).

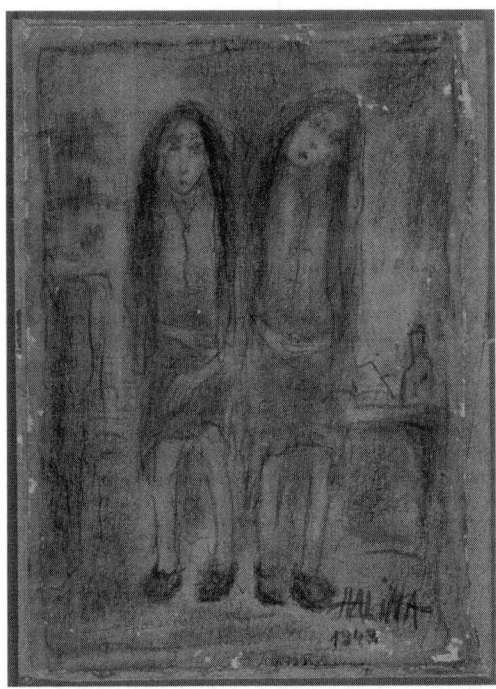

Figure 9.1 Halina Olomucki (1919–2007). *Two Women Hiding.* Warsaw ghetto, 1943.

The engagement between artist and sitter in the examples of portraits from camps and ghettos highlights the receptivity, emotion and connection that make up the experiential value. Perhaps the abundance of portraits created in camps and ghettos is due to the meaning that was found in their creation.

Another category of Holocaust artwork, landscape imagery, suggests an immersion in nature that is also characteristic of experiential values of meaning. Commentary from artists indicates that their landscape drawings and paintings were used as an opportunity to take in the natural beauty that they occasionally saw. Karl Schwesig (as cited in Sujo, 2001) described his desire to paint while he was interned at the Saint-Cyprien transit camp:

> One loaf of bread a day for nine people, no soap, no clean clothing, we can't sleep because of the fleas, we sleep on the earth, we have no cooking utensils (just a tin) or cutlery (just a wooden spoon). Degrading accommodation... I wish I had some watercolours to paint the impressive mountains and vineyards (p. 36).

Despite the "degrading accommodation" that Schwesig described—or perhaps because of its stark contrast to the natural beauty beyond the camp—the artist was able to recognize and appreciate nature, thus engaging in the experiential pathway toward meaning.

Attitudinal

The attitudinal value is often considered the most important in finding meaning, as it requires an individual to transcend their circumstances. This value refers to how one responds in an arduous situation that is outside their control and supports how meaning can be found in suffering. Explained Frankl:

> There is also purpose in that life which is almost barren of both creation and enjoyment and which admits of but one possibility of high moral behavior: namely, in man's attitude to his existence and existence restricted by external forces... Without suffering and death human life cannot be complete (2006, p. 106).

An individual can find meaning in the midst of suffering by how they choose to act in response to the situation causing such anguish. Wong (2014) elaborated on Frankl's writings, explaining that meaning can be found by taking a defiant attitude to confront suffering; finding a lesson within the experience; revising, rather than forgoing, goals, values and beliefs; and finding enjoyment and comfort within the experience of suffering. The attitudinal value involves choice, values and actions taken.

Examples of the attitudinal value in Holocaust art are numerous. The decision to make art indicated a choice in how one could live within the confines of their suffering. In their exploration of concentration camp art, Blatter and Milton (1981) wrote: "Ironically, the situation that reduced men and women to mere numbers also occasionally provided them with the opportunity to create" (p. 25). This statement illuminates the use of art making in response to adversity. When stripped of their safety and identity, some captives responded through art. And by choosing to create artwork, to respond in an authentic and genuine way, Holocaust artists demonstrated the attitudinal value of meaning. For Esther Lurie, for example, drawing was an initial and sustained response to the chaos she encountered in the Kovno ghetto

(USHMM, 2020). In an interview with Yad Vashem, surviving artist Alexander Bogen described his automatic response to seeing an orphaned girl in the ghetto:

> When I was in the ghetto, I saw a little girl with a doll standing next to a wall. I asked her where her parents were. They had already been taken to concentration camps and she was standing like that, not crying, and holding the doll's hand. And I, a man armed with a handgun and two grenades, a strong man, stood in front of that miserable creature, and I couldn't help. I felt very bad. I was a man and the feeling that you can't help this little girl... the only thing I could do... I took out my pencil and drew her, almost subconsciously (as cited in Jano and Sternin, n.d., para 8.)

What Bogen described was a situation beyond his control. Though he felt disempowered, he began drawing the girl (Figure 9.2), as that was the only way he could find to respond.

Bogen elaborated on his response to witnessing tragedy in the ghetto:

> But what compelled me to draw was reality. As far as I was concerned, there was no artistic thought, but a reaction to what happened in front of me. When you see something horrible you feel an electric current from your heart and you do this thing. You don't plan it (as cited in Jano and Sternin, n.d., para 8.)

Though Bogen did not specifically cite the attitudinal value, his description indicates that in that moment, when he was confronted with the reality of the Vilnius ghetto,

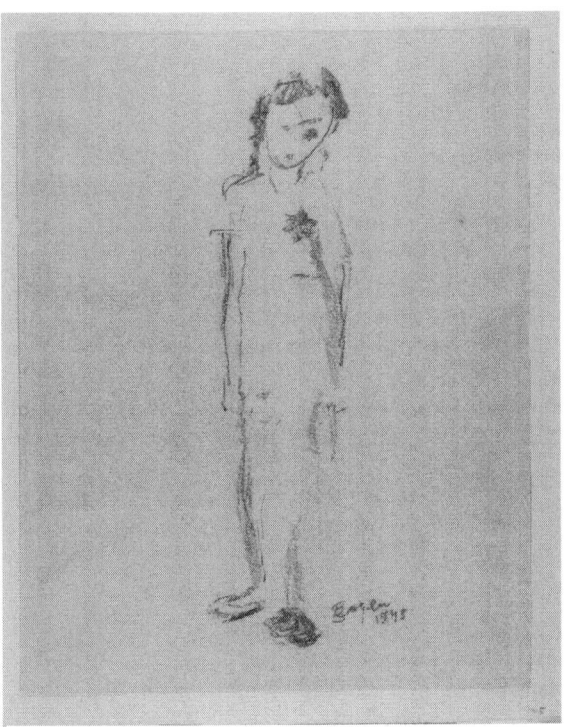

Figure 9.2 Alexander Bogen (b. 1916), *Girl with Jewish Badge*. Vilna ghetto, 1943. Charcoal on paper, 45.8 × 34.7 cm. Collection of the Yad Vashem Art Museum, Jerusalem. Gift of the artist. Photo © Yad Vashem Art Museum, Jerusalem

he was meant to draw. He felt compelled by an internal force to respond to the desperate situation in front of him. He found meaning by responding automatically, from the heart. By drawing, Bogen determined how he would confront the tragic reality of his situation. Doing so allowed him to evoke personal values and to respond authentically to the suffering that he was helpless to change.

The attitudinal value is also evidenced by the visual artists employed in Terezín, who risked relative comfort in order to speak their truth. Bedrich Fritta, Leo Hass, Otto Ungar and Felix Bloch worked as artists or designers prior to their deportation to the ghetto. Because of their known skills, they were employed to create propaganda and other artwork for Nazi use in the Terezín technical department. This assignment was comfortable and safe, relative to other positions in the ghetto: the artists worked indoors, so they were protected from harsh elements; and since they provided a useful service for their captors, their lives were considered worthy. However, the work they did was disingenuous, and they also wanted to document the realities of the ghetto. These artists were fully aware that unofficial artwork—especially images that contradicted their propaganda art—was prohibited; but they chose to make it anyway. When faced with a situation in which they had limited control and were surrounded by suffering, they decided to draw and paint what they actually experienced.

In his discussion of these artists, Langer stated:

> it is difficult to imagine what it must have been like for craftsman who were forced to spend their days falsifying their lives by pretending to engage freely in their chosen vocation, while secretly preparing a portfolio of death as their legacy (1995, pp. 666–667).

Indeed, the dissonance between their commissioned and clandestine works was likely difficult to reconcile. However, I believe that the clandestine works were necessary for the artists to create, in order to live and act in accordance with their values. This choice exemplifies the attitudinal value, as they decided how they wanted to respond to their horrific circumstances.

This value was also evident in my interview with Yehuda Bacon, who felt inclined to depict the details of the gas chambers and crematoria in drawings immediately following liberation. When faced with the magnitude of the genocide he witnessed, he made the decision to document what he could in order to be a voice for those who had perished (Y. Bacon, personal communication, September 26, 2017). This act is an embodiment of Wong's (2014) elaboration of the attitudinal value, which includes confronting tragedy and transforming suffering into an opportunity to be an example of strength to others.

THE VALUES TOWARD MEANING IN ART THERAPY

Frankl's three values, or principles, toward finding meaning were embedded in the act of creating artwork in Nazi camps and ghettos. Through creative, experiential, and attitudinal means, victim artists found meaning in the midst of suffering. The values that Frankl identified as pathways toward finding meaning are of particular relevance to art therapists, as our work includes each of these capacities. The creative value is inherent to art therapy practice. As Ottemiller and Awais (2016) note, an "essential component that art therapists bring is the inherent belief that everyone has the innate ability to create art" (p. 146). The act of creation—be it a small sketch or a large painting—can help our clients to find meaning, as their creative endeavor brings something new into existence.

The experiential principle toward meaning can be achieved in an art therapy session through engagement with the art materials, the image and the art therapist. The art experience is what leads to meaning, as the individual feels clay on their hands or a pencil between their fingers. The taking in of colors blending on a paper or the rhythmic process of moving a paintbrush across a canvas can evoke meaning, as the individual experiences these sensations. Connecting with their own artwork—or, in group art therapy, with the artwork of a peer—can also support finding meaning through experience, as the individual takes in and experiences the essence of the artwork in front of them. Moon (2016) noted that arts-based therapy groups allow individuals an opportunity to be witnessed with compassion and authenticity, both by the group leader and by peers. Individuals develop connections with peers and the art therapist by making art together and sharing a form of expression. This connection, through the witnessing and understanding of each other's expression, can lead to a deepened experience of meaning. As Moon explained, meaning is found in the context of interpersonal relationships (2016).

In conceptualizing the experiential value, I am reminded of the art therapy groups that I previously led on an inpatient psychiatric unit. At the end of each group, I always invited participants to share their artwork. After each individual had shared, I asked the other group members if anything in the artwork resonated with them. This was often the case and group members were able to recognize aspects of their own stories in their peers' work. The connection found within the art of another seemed to yield a deeper understanding of themselves. From this connection, group members were also often able to build interpersonal connections. In that moment, sharing artwork around a table, the sense of cohesive meaning that Heintzelman and King (2014) described was felt, as the dynamics between the group members, the environment and the art all suddenly made sense.

The term *attitudinal values* refers to the way in which a human responds to challenging or painful circumstances. Frankl asserted that even if an individual is unable to access meaning through the creative or experiential, they can find meaning in how they react to a challenging situation. The attitudinal principle of meaning is achieved first by choosing to go to art therapy in an attempt to address one's stressors or ailments. By choosing to see a therapist of any kind, an individual is making an effort to confront or change their situation. In seeking therapy, the individual shows a willingness to delve into their inner resources, search for inspiration and even connect with others who are suffering (Wong, 2012). The act of creating artwork in the face of adversity represents this value. This can be seen in a spectrum of art therapy practices, from clinical to community work.

Art making is an intentional process full of choices. The artist must select materials to use and a subject to depict, and mobilize the confidence to externalize their inner experience. I recently met with a 25-year-old female client whom I have been seeing for almost seven years. She has struggled with anorexia and depression since early adolescence and has spent the majority of the past year in residential treatment centers. Despite our long therapeutic relationship, she rarely made art in our sessions. Upon returning to outpatient therapy, I suggested that we make art together, which she begrudgingly agreed to do. I offered different two-dimensional materials and she chose to paint with watercolors on a small sheet of paper. I reminded her that I would not be judging or grading her artwork; and that the goal was simply to modulate her anxiety, which had been particularly high. She struggled to begin, but eventually painted abstractly on her paper while we talked about her week. As she painted, I noticed a shift in her affect. For years, our conversations had centered on her identity as an anorexic. She could easily share stories about the people she met in treatment; or one of the times she required a feeding tube; or the limited support she received from her family. But as she painted, she appeared to take ownership and responsibility over the events in her life. She spoke passionately about returning to college and elaborated on the hurt she felt from her family members "who don't expect anything else from me." Although I had worked with her for almost a decade, I had rarely witnessed this impassioned side of her. So often, she presented as defeated; as if she didn't expect any therapeutic interventions to result in substantial change. Engaging in the artistic process seemed to ignite a previously dormant spark in her. Instead of engaging in our session as someone suffering from anorexia, she showed a desire and capacity to recover from her disorder.

I think the decision making inherent in painting showed this young woman that she had a degree of autonomy and freedom. For years, she—as well as her family members—had viewed her diagnosis as something she suffered from. As such, she had given up on her ability to change her situation. However, in that session, she recognized a capacity to make a change. By agreeing to paint, she made a decision to act differently, priming herself to consider an alternative response to her pain. In painting, she recognized and acted on her own capacity to respond, instead of just enduring.

She played with the colors and eventually painted a flower. She seemed guarded and uncertain, but kept painting and kept talking. I noticed that she wrote out the name of her niece and in that moment, I saw her will for meaning. Two months prior, this client had attempted suicide. She reported that as she almost blacked out, she heard her niece's voice and knew she had to survive. Once again, her niece had manifested a presence, and I saw that as a found meaning. We both knew that her niece was important to her; but to write out the name in her painting further reinforced the meaning her niece offered. This client continues to struggle. However, she is more readily open to making art in sessions and recognizes the shift in her affect when she does. My hope is to continue emboldening her to find meaning and take responsibility in fighting her illness, instead of living passively with it. Explained Wong:

> To choose the possibilities for change is to live an authentic life and become fully human. On the other hand, when individuals avoid the risk of change and choose to remain where they are, then they are living an inauthentic existence (2005, p.7).

By painting, this client took a risk and engaged differently in our session. In doing so, she expressed an authentic side of herself that was often silenced by her illness. This led her to engage as a human, and not as the disorder that has defined so much of her life.

SELF-TRANSCENDENCE

Meaning is found when we experience our world through investment in our values (Dubois, 2004), which involves external factors. This requires self-transcendence: the act of looking beyond ourselves. Self-transcendence is achieved when one shifts their focus from personal needs to a place of concern for another human, animal, cause or value. Frankl asserted that self-transcendence is an innate part of humanity, as we are always pointed or directed to something other than ourselves (1966). He continued: "being human profoundly means to be open to the world, a world, that is, which is replete with other beings to encounter and with meanings to fulfill" (p. 97). Vesely Frankl described self-transcendence as similar to the human eye: always being directed at something outside of ourselves (A. Vesely Frankl, personal communication, November 18, 2021). The very concept of self-transcendence contradicts the Freudian pleasure principle and the homeostasis principle (Fletcher, 1942), both of which place emphasis on achieving personal happiness and ultimately restoring an internal equilibrium. Frankl lauded Charlotte Buhler, who argued that the basic hypothesis of psychodynamic theory is self-satisfaction (1965). Like Frankl, Buhler argued that pleasure and satisfaction are secondary gains to living a meaningful life. Humans pose "a primary, or native orientation, in the direction of creating and of values" (Buhler, 1965, p. 55); and therefore, psychotherapy should be oriented to this inherent characteristic of human nature. Happiness and pleasure should be viewed in a larger context, such as *the reason* an individual feels happiness, pleasure and satisfaction (Frankl, 1966). In logotherapy, it is the therapist's job to help clients find meaning in the greater context of their world.

Although the art-making process is a personal one, it is fundamentally self-transcendent. To create art is to express one's feelings to an outside audience. In art therapy, the client is encouraged to create a representation of their internal experience. The simple process of bringing one's inner experience into their external world is an example of self-transcendence, as they surpass the boundary of self. Moon explained that "art making engages the clients in a world outside of themselves" (2016, p. 155). The process of reflecting on a piece of artwork supports self-transcendence, as the client is forced to see the artwork in front of them, instead of inside them. Describing their piece to the art therapist, or to peers in a group, bridges a connection with others, forcing the client to interact outside of themselves. Moon (2016) articulated that art making within a group represents an offering to life.

In defining self-transcendence in art making, I am reminded of the Holocaust artists working individually and in creative communities, committing to a goal larger than themselves. While they knew their actions were potentially dangerous, they felt compelled by a greater cause. Self-transcendence is evident in the commitment to document the realities of camp and ghetto life, and the pain of others. It can be found in the desire to connect with another, despite one's own pain and suffering. It is seen in the tenacity of hope that their artworks would be found and witnessed. The act of self-transcendence is seen in the way art making allowed these artists to psychologically evade danger by performing something familiar and comfortable.

Zofia Stępień-Bator's drawing of a female prisoner praying below an imagined Virgin Mary (Figure 9.3) is a strong example of self-transcendence in Holocaust art. The fact that the soft, comforting image was created in Auschwitz shows the artist's ability to transcend her reality. Stępień-Bator was known to draw idealized portraits of fellow prisoners in Auschwitz in a conscious attempt to beautify the ugliness, transcending her subjects from prisoners into the women they once were. Additionally, Stępień-Bator's drawing indicates a sense of hope and commitment to a cause—in

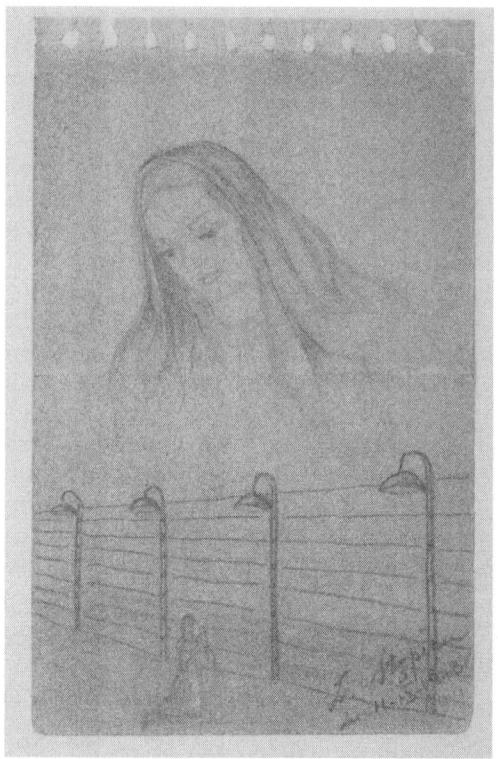

Figure 9.3 Zofia Stępień-Bator. *Prayer.* Auschwitz 1943. Collections of the Auschwitz-Birkenau State Museum.

this case, religion—beyond herself. The crouched figure appears to have found a small space to think outside of her deplorable reality, and to experience hope and faith in something both literally and figuratively larger than herself.

FREEDOM AND RESPONSIBILITY

Logotherapy sees the individual as responsible for finding their meaning in life. Responsibility is realized through free will, which Yalom viewed as an existential concern. The reality that humans have the freedom to make life choices places great responsibility on us. Artists working in camps and ghettos took on this responsibility, recognizing it as a rare opportunity to exercise their freedom of choice. The decision to pick up a pencil or stub of charcoal and make art, even clandestinely, can be viewed as a function of free will. Opportunities to act on free will were limited in the constraints of ghettos and camps. Those targeted in the Holocaust were barred from the luxury of choice, as they had been uprooted from their previous lives and forced into deplorable conditions. They witnessed and endured suffering with little, if any, ability to protect themselves or others. Death camps in particular were "designed to diminish and annihilate one's freedom of choice and sense of responsibility" (Davidov & Eisikovits, 2015, p. 88). Considering this experience of complete powerlessness, one can surmise the appeal of artistic creation regardless of the known risks. Creativity allowed for decision making, which Davidov and Eisikovits (2015) argued was crucial in avoiding *muselmann* status. The capacity for decision making strengthened the spirit, as it represented a degree of hope and will. Frankl (1959, 2006) argued that in any situation, individuals have a choice in their existence. The act of drawing or painting represented a choice, a conscious resolution to act; and therefore, as in the case of Halina Olomucki, it delivered a motivation to survive (M.Alon, personal communication, September 25, 2017). Ultimately, making art was a choice of how to live one's life in the context of the Holocaust.

Fabry related responsibility and free will to art making through the analogy of a blank canvas (1987). An art professor noticed that his students panicked when faced with an empty canvas on an easel. The students were accustomed to being given a specific assignment or commission and, having no direction, experienced an existential challenge. They didn't know what was expected of them without guidelines to follow or paramaters to stay within. Fabry used this analogy to illustrate the existential crisis of choice. Without concrete rules, humans can feel at a loss with regard to how to guide themselves. I remember feeling this in the spring of my senior year of college. For my entire life, I had followed a specific path, from grade school to high school to college. I had always been on the same trajectory as my peers; and though I made decisions based on my own abilities, values and interests, I always knew what the next step would be. It dawned on me that my decisions after graduation would be completely my own; that there was no set path to follow. My peers would be moving in different directions, and I recognized the responsibility I had to forge my own path moving forward. I remember the fear I felt in knowing that I was solely responsible, and that I would progress in a direction that was specific to me. It was exciting and liberating, but also terrifying.

Fabry's analogy alludes to the responsibility inherent in art making. Art therapists are familiar with clients feeling overwhelmed or discouraged by a blank sheet of paper, canvas or slab of clay. While some clients can jump right into the art process, others struggle when given freedom of creativity. Though scary, for both the client and the art therapist, this confrontation with responsibility is an opportunity to help the client find their spiritual, noetic dimension. The client can be reminded that while the burden of responsibility is present, there is also an opportunity to find meaning. This can be used as a metaphor for making authentic choices and developing a sense of responsibility over one's life. The art therapist can be present with the client in the moment of fear and help them to access their inner resources. For example, if a client does not know where to start, I will suggest they begin with their favorite color; or if they are feeling angry, perhaps their least favorite color. I will suggest finding a magazine image that reminds them of a certain person or memory and begin a collage based on that. If they are experiencing a conflict, I might encourage them to split their paper in half and assign each side to their conflicting thoughts. I have told clients they can rip up their paper if they are not content with what they made, which no one has ever done—at least, not without greater context. I think having that option shows clients that the choices they make on the paper don't have to be permanent, but are merely one small step in a potentially new direction. I remind them that while they may feel uncertain and out of control in other areas, they have complete control over their artwork, which can be seen as a burden and a privilege. I am reminded of Frederick Terna, who found that the white rectangle of paper he obtained in Terezín was a unique opportunity to assert control. While all freedoms were taken away from him, he found a sense of autonomy in making art. Though I rarely share that exact example, I use it to help guide my clients toward making their first mark and taking the responsibility to do so.

As Fabry eloquently stated: "our human spirit supplies the resources through which health may be restored and maintained" (1987, p. 18). While art therapy involves physical and cognitive abilities, our clients' artwork is sourced from the spiritual dimension. This unique aspect of humanity is what logotherapy serves to foster: to help individuals find meaning and live authentically. An authentic existence occurs when an individual's actions are aligned with their values and potential (Frankl, 1967; Ortiz & Florez, 2015). The concept of authenticity in art therapy dates back to Cane (1951), who led her students to engage with their authentic imagery. Nothing is more authentic than one's artistic expression. A logotherapeutic art therapy process is one that encourages authentic expression to help clients identify personal meaning and values. Through art making, they can practice taking responsibility and eventually make life choices that are congruent with their values, allowing them to find meaning. Art therapists know that the creative process can lead an individual to find meaning. We are aware of the renewed sense of accomplishment, hope, release and awareness that art making offers. Logotherapy provides a framework for us to understand how the creative process facilitates the finding of meaning.

Viktor Frankl first conceived of logotherapy as a physician in Vienna in 1926. His experiences in Terezín, Auschwitz and Dachau only strengthened his resolve that meaning is paramount to existence. He spent his career elucidating his philosophy and brought about a change to the then dominant fields of psychology. It is beyond my scope in this chapter to fully deconstruct and critique logotherapy. My aim was to describe key elements of logotherapy as they pertain to art making, in order to fuse logotherapy philosophy with art therapy theory and practice. My research on the art of the Holocaust has illuminated how individuals found meaning through creativity in abhorrent conditions. If individuals in the midst of a genocide were able to find meaning through art, I believe that art therapy clients in contemporary practices can do the same. By integrating logotherapy with art therapy, I hope that art therapists can support their clients' search for meaning.

REFERENCES

Ameli, M. (2016). Integrating logotherapy with cognitive behavior therapy: a worthy challenge. In *Logotherapy and Existential Analysis*. Cham, Switzerland: Springer, pp. 197–217.

Amishai-Maisels, Z. (1993). *Depiction and interpretation: The influence of the Holocaust on visual arts.* Tarrytown, NY: Pergamon Press.

Betensky, M. (2001). Phenomenological art therapy. In J. A. Rubin (ed.). *Approaches to art therapy: Theory and technique* (2nd ed.). New York, NY: Routledge, pp. 121–133.

Blatner, J. & Milton, S. (1981). *Art of the Holocaust.* New York, NY: Routledge.

Buhler, C. (1965). Some observations on the psychology of the third force. *Journal of Humanistic Psychology*, 5, 54.

Cane, F. (1951). *The artist in each of us.* New York, NY: Pantheon.

Costanza, M. (1982). *The living witness: Art in the concentration camps and ghettos.* New York, NY: The Free Press.

Dalek, J. & Swiebocka, T. (1989). *Suffering and hope: Artistic creations of the Oświęcim prisoners.* Trans. Jolanta Kosiec. Oświęcim, Poland: Panstwowe Muzeum Auschwitz-Birkenau.

Davidov, J. & Eisikovits, Z. (2015). Free will in total institutions: The case of choice inside Nazi death camps. *Consciousness and Cognition, 34,* 87–97. doi: 10.1016/j.concog.2015.03.018

Dissanayake, E. (1995). *Homo aestheticus: Where art comes from and why.* Seattle, WA: University of Washington Press.

Ernzen, F. I. (1990). Frankl's Mountain Range Exercise: A logotherapy activity for small groups. *International Forum for Logotherapy, 13*(2), 133–134.

Fabry, J. B. (1987). *The Pursuit of meaning: Viktor Frank, logotherapy, and life.* Berkeley, CA: Institute of Logotherapy Press.

Fenner, P. (2012). What do we see? Extending understanding of visual experience in the art therapy encounter. *Art Therapy, 29*(1), 11–18.

Fletcher, J. M. (1942). Homeostasis as an explanatory principle in psychology. *Psychological Review, 49*(1), 80–87. https://doi.org/10.1037/h0058280

Frankl, V. (1959/2006). *Man's search for meaning* (5th ed.) (I. Lasch, trans.). Boston, MA: Beacon Press.

Frankl, V. E. (1966). Self-transcendence as a human phenomenon. *Journal of Humanistic Psychology, 6*(2), 97–106.

Frankl, V. (1967). *Psychotherapy and existentialism: Selected papers on logotherapy.* New York, NY: Simon and Schuster.

Frankl, V. (1973). *The doctor and the soul. From psychotherapy to logotherapy.* New York, NY: Vintage Books.

Frankl, V. E. (1988). *The will to meaning: Foundations and applications of logotherapy.* New York, NY: Meridian

Heintzelman, S. J. & King, L. A. (2014). (The feeling of) Meaning-as-information. *Personality and Social Psychology Review,* 18, 153–167.

Jano, M. and Sternin, M. (n.d.) *Interview with Alexander Bogen, survivor and artist.* https://www.yadvashem.org/articles/interviews/alexander-bogen.html

Juni, S. (2016). Survivor guilt: A critical review from the lens of the Holocaust. *International Review of Victimology, 22*(3), 321–337.

Kantor, A. (1971). *The book of Alfred Kantor: An artist's journal of the Holocaust.* New York, NY: McGraw Hill.

Kaimal, G. (2019) Adaptive Response Theory: An evolutionary framework for clinical research in art therapy. *Art Therapy, 36*(4), 215–219. doi: 10.1080/07421656.2019.1667670

Kellermann, N. P. (2001). The long-term psychological effects and treatment of Holocaust trauma. *Journal of Loss & Trauma, 6*(3), 197–218.

Lamberti, M. (1995). Making art in the Terezín concentration camp. *New England Review (1990), 17*(4), 104–111.

Langer, L. (1996). *Admitting the Holocaust: Collected essays.* New York, NY: Oxford University Press.

Lantz, J. (1993). *Existential family therapy: Using the concepts of Viktor Frankl.* Northvale, NJ: Jason Aronson.

Leclerc, J. (2011). Re-presenting trauma: The witness function in the art of the Holocaust. *Art Therapy, 28*(2), 82–89. doi: 10.1080/07421656.2011.580181.

May, R. (1975). *The courage to create.* New York, NY: Norton.

Melton, A. M. & Schulenberg, S. E. (2008). On the measurement of meaning: Logotherapy's empirical contributions to humanistic psychology. *The Humanistic Psychologist, 36*(1), 31–44.

Moon, B. (2009). *Existential art therapy: The canvas mirror.* Springfield, IL: Charles C. Thomas.

Moon, B. L. (2016). *Art-based group therapy: Theory and practice.* Springfield, IL: Charles C. Thomas.

Moreh-Rosenberg, E. (2016). *The art from the Holocaust*. Cologne, Germany: Wienand Verlag.

Ortiz, E. M. & Flórez, I. A. (2016). Meaning-centered psychotherapy: A Socratic clinical practice. In S. S. Schulenberg (ed.). *Clarifying and furthering existential psychotherapy: Theories, methods, and practices*. Cham, Switzerland: Springer International, pp. 59–78.

Ottemiller, D. D. & Awais, Y. J. (2016). A model for art therapists in community-based practice. *Art Therapy, 33*(3), 144–150.

Pfeifer, E. (2021). Logotherapy, existential analysis, music therapy: Theory and practice of meaning-oriented music therapy. *The Arts in Psychotherapy, 72*, 101730.

Purjo, T. (2013). On interpreting terms used in logotherapy and existential analysis. In *International Forum for Logotherapy, 36*, 16–20.

Sharp, W. G., Wilson, K. G. & Schulenberg, S. E. (2004). Use of paradoxical intention in the context of Acceptance and Commitment Therapy. *Psychological Reports, 95*(3), 946–948.

Schneider, K. J. & Krug, O. T. (2017). *Existential-humanistic therapy*. Washington, DC: American Psychological Association.

Schulenberg, S. E. (2003). Empirical research and logotherapy. *Psychological Reports, 93*(1), 307–319.

Schulenberg, S. E. (2004). Expanding the topography: Variations on Frankl's Mountain Range Exercise. *International Forum for Logotherapy, 27*(2), 80–83.

Schulenberg, S. E., Hutzell, R. R., Nassif, C. & Rogina, J. M. (2008). Logotherapy for clinical practice. *Psychotherapy, 45*(4), 447–463. doi: 10.1037/a0014331

Sieradzka, A. (2019). *Art at Auschwitz*. http://lekcja.auschwitz.org/en_18_sztuka/ Oświęcim: Państwowe Muzeum Auschwitz-Birkenau/Auschwitz-Birkenau State Museum

Sujo, G. (2001). *Legacies of silence: The visual arts and Holocaust memory*. London, England: Philip Wilson Publishers.

Thir, M. & Batthyány, A. (2016). The state of empirical research on logotherapy and existential analysis. In *Logotherapy and existential analysis*. Cham, Switzerland: Springer, pp. 53–74.

Tomić, I., Milić, V., Lazić, D. and Marinković, S. (2019). Psychological survival in Banjica concentration camp due to inmate creativity. A recommendation to future victims. *Austin Anthropology, 3*(2), 1008.

United States Holocaust Memorial Museum (2020). *Esther Lurie*. Adapted from United States Holocaust Memorial Museum, and United States Holocaust Memorial Council (1997). *Hidden History of the Kovno Ghetto*. Boston, MA: Little, Brown and Co., pp. 168–171.

Wilkinson, R. A. & Chilton, G. (2018). *Positive art therapy theory and practice: Integrating positive psychology with art therapy*. New York, NY: Routledge.

Wong, P. T. (2005). Existential and humanistic theories. In J. C. Thomas & D. L. Segal (eds.). *Comprehensive handbook of personality and psychopathology*. Hoboken, NJ: John Wiley & Sons, Inc., pp.192–211.

Wong, P. T. (2009). Meaning therapy: An integrative and positive existential psychotherapy. *Journal of Contemporary Psychotherapy, 40*(2), 85–93. doi: 10.1007/s10879-009-9132-6

Wong, P. T. (2012). *The human quest for meaning: Theories, research, and applications*, 2nd ed. New York, NY: Routledge.

Wong, P. T., & Wong, L. C. (2013). A meaning-centered approach to building youth resilience. In *The human quest for meaning*. New York, NY: Routledge, pp. 631–664.

Wong, P. T. P. (2014). Viktor Frankl's meaning seeking model and positive psychology. In A. Batthyany & P. Russo Netzer (eds.). *Meaning in existential and positive psychology*. New York, NY: Springer

Yad Vashem. *The pen and the sword: Jewish artist and partisan Alexander Bogen*. http://www.yadvashem.org/yv/en/exhibitions/bogen/about.asp.

Yad Vashem. *Interview with Alexander Bogen, survivor and artist*. https://www.yadvashem.org/articles/interviews/alexander-bogen.html.

CHAPTER 10

ART LOGOTHERAPY IN PRACTICE

I began my doctoral research on the art of the Holocaust in the hope that it would inform my clinical practice. At the time, I did not view myself as a researcher or as an academic. The thought of pursuing a terminal degree in art therapy never crossed my mind until I learned about the practitioner-based research doctoral program at Mount Mary University. I was attracted to the idea of research being executed by practitioners and excited at the prospect of expanding my existing knowledge of Holocaust artwork. Since the subject of Holocaust art had long been integrated into my personal knowledge of art therapy, I anticipated that a deeper dive into the phenomenon could further support my clinical work. In a 1977 critique of academia, Idinopolus wrote that "striving for disciplined knowledge of one area of experience is not enough; what more is required is that the specialized knowledge be extended to achieve insight into other areas of experience" (p. 410). Though the institutions under his critique have evolved since his article was published, Indinopolus's words resonated with my own integration of research and practice. As intended, the research I conducted in one niche discipline has given me insight into another. My study of Holocaust art continues to inform my art therapy practice today.

The study of Holocaust art has supported a logotherapeutic framework that I incorporate into my clinical work. That is, the emphasis of my practice involves guiding my clients to identify meaning. I do this by focusing my attention on the spiritual or noetic dimension, rather than on the pathology that my clients present. Though I consider the physical and psychological issues at hand, and refer to higher levels of care if these areas require more specialized medical attention, my goal is to work with clients within the realm of the spiritual dimension to help them find meaning. According to existential thought, a sense of meaning is essential for persevering through hardship (Frankl, 1959/2006, 2004; Schulenberg, Hutzell, Nassif & Rogina, 2008). The discovery of meaning from adversity or suffering is what I strive to help my clients achieve. Many individuals have experienced life events that have impacted their current daily functioning and their existence as a whole. Even though it cannot change their past experiences or their current realities, art therapy can guide them to access and bolster their spiritual dimension in the face of adversity. To retain a sense of humanity and to facilitate spiritual growth, I aim to help my clients accept and realign themselves with the unstable, often painful aspects of their existence (Schneider, 2015).

The goal in existentially oriented therapy is not to ameliorate a condition, but rather to help people "develop a new relationship to a shocking part of themselves" (Schneider, 2015, p. 22) in order to continue living within painful circumstances. Likewise, contemporary logotherapy "fulfills clients' needs to comprehend, to make sense, to reconstruct the general vision of the world, to have an orientation, to realize their potential, to reach authentic living" (Leontiev, 2016, p. 284). Accordingly, the client is encouraged to accept their new position by developing a willingness to

DOI: 10.4324/9781003160885-14

continue living within their changed life construct. Meaning is what supports this willingness. As seen through the examples of artists working in Nazi camps and ghettos, art making can lead an individual to find meaning in suffering. The creative process can bring an individual into a contemplative state which may evoke one or more of several positive responses: an affirmation of existence; a connection to others; a feeling of hope and comfort; a sense of autonomy and responsibility; and an opportunity for self-transcendence. Through this process, individuals can begin to find meaning within their life experience, which makes the new reality of their existence more tolerable.

Logotherapy was originally positioned to supplement traditional psychotherapy (Costello, 2016; Southwick, Lowthert & Graber, 2016), and often has been considered ancillary to other therapeutic philosophies and modalities (Leontiev, 2016). Despite this intention, logotherapy has gained momentum as clinicians aim for a humanistic approach that they can tailor to clients' individual needs. Rogina (2015) coined the term *noetic activation* to describe his method of logotherapeutic practice, through which he aims to reignite an individual's search for meaning through personal values, strengths and relationships.

Frankl (2014) observed that "psychotherapy endeavors to bring instinctual facts to consciousness," whereas logotherapy "seeks to bring to awareness the spiritual realities" (p. 43). Although psychotherapy has evolved in the years since Frankl's original writings, his clarification remains relevant—especially in the US healthcare system, which is geared toward symptom amelioration rather than spiritual growth. In the previous chapter, I proposed similarities between art therapy and logotherapy to suggest an integration of logotherapy philosophy into art therapy theory and practice. I will use this final chapter to share case vignettes from my clinical practice illustrating how I have incorporated the findings of my research into a meaning-based approach. For context, I must first provide information about my practice. I currently work as a sole practitioner in Annapolis, Maryland, seeing mostly adolescents and young adults. The majority of my clients carry an eating disorder diagnosis and are often referred to me from an intensive treatment program. Such disorders are often accompanied by depression, anxiety, and self-injurious behaviors. Some of my clients have experienced traumatic events and a few struggle with ongoing PTSD symptoms. They are predominantly white females between the ages of 12 and 45 who are in high school, college or graduate school; or who work full time. I estimate that 80% of my caseload utilizes their health insurance, while the other 20% is self-pay—either at my full rate or on a sliding scale. My clients live in central Maryland, in the Baltimore, Washington, and Annapolis metropolitan areas.

Each of the case examples that I share in this chapter could be viewed through a psychodynamic or trauma-focused lens, or an entirely different philosophy. However, my intention is to demonstrate how a logotherapeutic approach can be incorporated into art therapy by mobilizing the inherent qualities of an individual (Graber, 2004) to promote wellbeing. I have organized these cases according to the themes that arose in my phenomenological study—witnessing, identity, hope, affirmation of existence, resilience, comfort, and connection—though there are certainly thematic overlaps between cases. I conclude by sharing two non-clinical examples which also demonstrate the finding of meaning through art making.

CASE VIGNETTES

Witnessing

The need to serve as a witness was a common motivator for artists creating in captivity across Europe (Leclerc, 2011). Artists working in the Holocaust held the dual role of victim and witness. They experienced their own ongoing suffering while simultaneously witnessing others experience the same. Some of the artists I spoke to felt the need to document what they had witnessed, especially since they had survived the suffering while others had not.

Although the clients in my practice have not witnessed the same degree of destruction, some have expressed a similar sense of burden from what they have both witnessed and endured. An example is the case of Kelly (pseudonym), a white 20-year-old woman who came to art therapy one year after leaving an abusive relationship. Kelly presented as driven and bright; at the time of treatment, she was a freshman in community college and planned to transfer to the University of Maryland to study biology. She said that her abuser had isolated her from friends and family; but in the past year since their breakup, she had reconnected with her friend group and was spending more time with her parents and brother. She felt optimistic about the future and had even started dating again.

Despite the bright spot she was in at the time of our sessions, Kelly continued to feel a sense of burden from the relationship. She did not report flashbacks, hypervigilance, nightmares or any other typical symptoms associated with PTSD. However, she described feeling haunted by memories of the abuse. She was disappointed in herself for staying in the relationship for as long as she did and alarmed at the realization that many women remain in such relationships for longer. Kelly was struck by the reality that others experience similar suffering and became increasingly concerned for other women in abusive relationships.

In one of our sessions, Kelly painted a large, wide-open eye surrounded by shades of blue and purple (Figure 10.1). She explained that the eye represented her "watching all of these things happen to me and not doing anything." A trauma-focused therapist might suggest that this painting was a depiction of dissociation, given Kelly's explanation of *watching herself*, in addition to her traumatic history. However, viewed in the context of logotherapy, the image presented as an example of self-distancing and self-transcendence. Kelly could position herself as a witness rather than a victim. She was able to conceptualize herself apart from her experience of abuse and recognize that she did not have to be abused again.

Kelly's struggle seemed to be about the burden of the witness. While painting, she discussed how overwhelmed she felt knowing that abusive relationships were not uncommon. Her words resonated with the burden of her witnessing. The painting of an eye was not solely about her experiences being abused; it also conveyed how she was helpless to do anything but watch as her reality crumbled. The painting suggested that her experience had opened her own eyes to the prevalence of domestic abuse. She was able to self-transcend and recognize that other women suffer similar experiences.

Kelly contacted me after we had terminated our therapeutic relationship. She shared that in her junior year, she had taken on a leadership role within her university's student mental health organization. She said that her work in art therapy

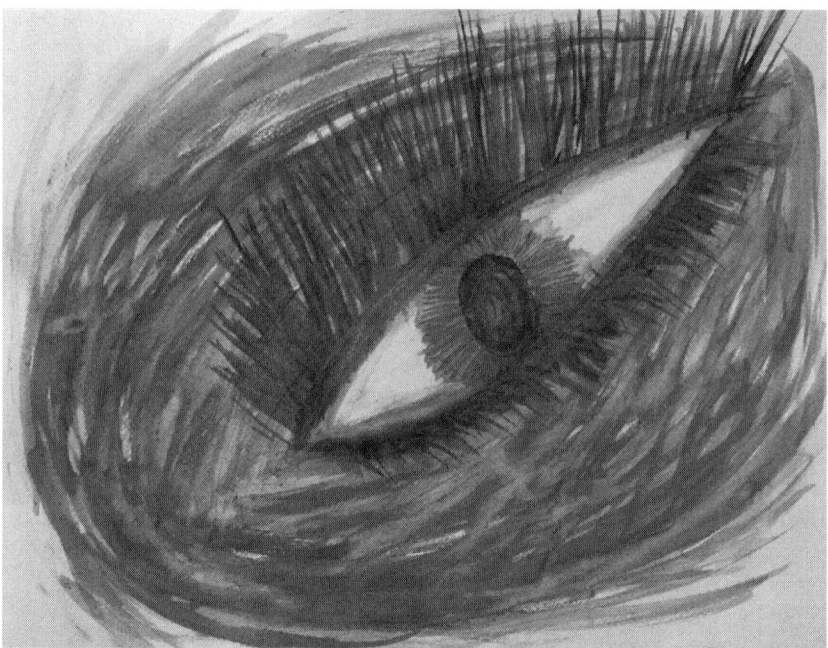

Figure 10.1 Witnessing, 2017. Watercolor on paper.

had "pushed [her] to take action and make a difference" (personal communication, 2018). Serving as an advocate for others, Kelly is exemplifying Frankl's will to meaning, in which an individual recognizes a particular role for themselves that makes use of their distinctive talents, characteristics and life experiences (Wong, 2014). Rather than let the abuse limit her to the status of a victim, she chose an attitude of defiance and was able to transcend her powerless experience as a victim to adopt a role of advocacy for others. Through art making, Kelly was able to rise above the weakness she felt as a victim of abuse and view herself as a survivor.

Identity

Creating artwork within Nazi ghettos and camp systems allowed individuals to transcend their prisoner identity, even briefly, to retain a sense of who they were prior to captivity (Amishai-Maisels, 1993). Spenser (2001) wrote that the artists creating within the Holocaust had an "important role, which was to deal with questions of identity and the need to perpetuate the continuity between the past and future" (p. 55). In creating, artists were able to reconnect with their authentic self and bolster their sense of identity. This theme was consistent in both my literature review and my study. In my clinical experience, I have seen that a profound loss of identity is also common to psychiatric patients. Clients may enter therapy feeling more aligned to their psychiatric symptoms than their authentic self (Morris & Willis-Rauch, 2011). Mental illness is frequently stigmatized and those who struggle can become consumed by the label of their diagnosis (Overton & Medina, 2008). I have worked with clients who can easily rattle off a list of their symptomatic behaviors but struggle to define themselves outside of their diagnosis. To counter this identity, I attempt to guide my clients to reconstruct their sense of self. As Kapitan (2009) described, art can be a liberating force that demands recognition of, and confrontation with, the very existence of one's self. In so doing, a sense of identity can emerge as separate from a client's diagnosis.

I have observed that for clients with eating disorders, there is a definite struggle to identify themselves apart from their disorder, as it has consumed them not just emotionally, but also physically. Since logotherapy emphasizes an individual's unique characteristics, it is a useful model in helping clients reconstruct their sense of identity as separate from the disorder. In this vein, I asked my client Molly (pseudonym) to create two portraits: one of herself and the other of her disorder. Using magazine images, she collaged a full portrait of her disorder, leaving very little empty space on the page. In contrast, the portrait of herself was almost completely blank. She admitted that she struggled to see herself as anything other than an anorexic.

I made Molly's collage accessible to her during each subsequent session. Whenever our work led her to identify a characteristic that was specific to herself, as opposed to her disorder, I asked her to represent it in some way on her collage. For example, when discussing her college classes, Molly mentioned that although she had been attached to the idea of earning a science degree, she was genuinely enjoying a particular class that led her to consider switching majors to a humanities field. She admitted that she had never felt passionate about her science classes, but pursued that major because it felt high-achieving and therefore admirable. The perfectionism that drove her disorder also influenced her initial choice of major as something she felt she had to do. I pointed out that her new area of interest was an example of an authentic part of her, something unrelated to her anorexia. Eventually, Molly's self-portrait became a mixed-media piece filled with imagery that comprised her non-disordered identity. She recognized her unique qualities and was able to see in her artwork that she was far more than her disorder and had an existence outside of it.

Affirmation of Existence

The Holocaust survivors I interviewed faced death, and the threat of death, on a daily basis. They described their existence within a camp or ghetto as tenuous—a stance that has been echoed in literature. Although the clients in my practice are not regularly confronted with the threat of death, many question the quality—and often the very point—of their existence. An adolescent client, Allie (pseudonym), came to art therapy one afternoon preoccupied with what she described as a "chair left on the side of the road." She explained that she had seen the chair—a discarded piece of furniture on a curb, waiting to be hauled away—and couldn't stop thinking about it. She wondered out loud if others would ever want it and became increasingly worried that it would get damaged in the thunderstorm that was forecast, rendering it even less desirable.

I suggested that she paint the chair because it appeared to be meaningful to her. As she painted the image of the abandoned chair (Figure 10.2), Allie began to understand her preoccupation with it. She admitted that she occasionally felt insecure in her peer and family relationships. She worried about her own existence and whether others viewed her as someone "worth salvaging," or whether she too would be "left out in the rain" someday.

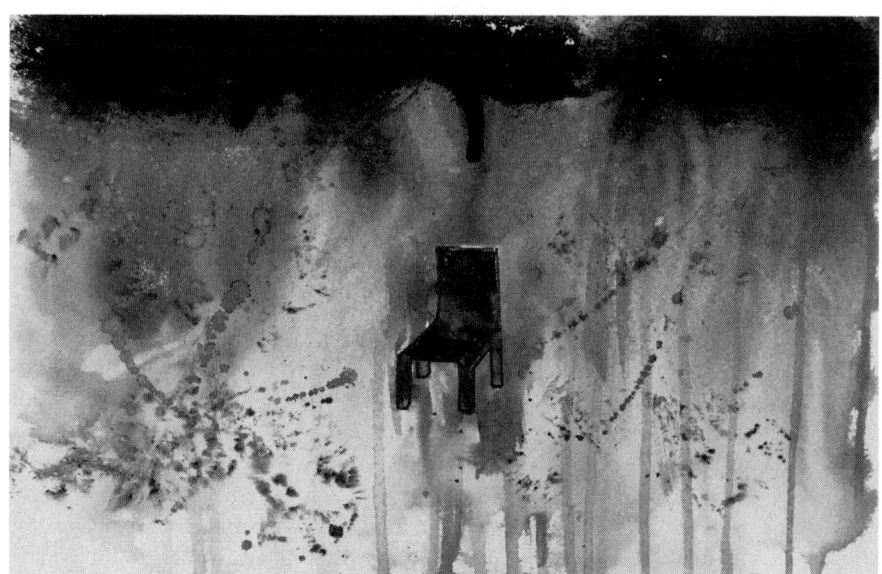

Figure 10.2 Discarded Chair, 2016. Watercolor and watercolor pigment on paper.

In her painting, Allie confronted what Sousa (2015) described as the *dimensions of existence.* Although there was substantial evidence that she was loved and highly regarded by the people in her life, Allie felt insignificant and questioned the value of her existence. She contemplated her life's purpose and whether she had the potential to find meaning or to discover that her existence was disposable. Although non-existentially oriented therapists might view Allie's concerns primarily as a symptom of depression, I acknowledged for her the paradox that is part of the existential exploration (Reker, 2000) through which she might ponder her capacity for meaning. By painting the imagery of the chair and talking about what resonated in it for her, Allie was able to engage in an art process that facilitated contemplation of her worries rather than pathologize her fears. She later acknowledged that since she had noticed and appreciated the chair, it was likely that others noticed and appreciated her.

Comfort

One of the most surprising aspects of Holocaust artwork is the abundance of bright and light-hearted images. Amalie Seckbach, for example, painted watercolors of flowers and surreal landscapes in Terezín which Rosenberg (2009) noted were contradictory to the reality of the ghetto. Dicker-Brandeis encouraged children to depict beauty from memory or their imagination, to counter their bleak environment (Makarova, 2001; Monnig, 2014; Wix, 2009). Some artists seemed motivated to draw in order to comfort themselves with memories of a better life. Testimony from survivor Judy Godos-Jacobs supports this assertion, as she recalled the bright subject matter of her artwork contrasting with the abysmal environment of the Bergen-Belsen camp, stating that her drawings were a reminder of the vibrant life she had once lived (personal communication, 2017). I was reminded of these brighter works when a 24-year-old female client, Elissa (pseudonym), wanted to draw Olaf the Snowman, a Disney character, in one of our sessions. Her desire initially seemed odd to me, as I thought that an animated snowman seemed regressive for a woman in her 20s and was incongruent with the heavy topics she usually discussed while she drew. Elissa had recently visited her hometown in New England and spoke about how disappointing the trip had been. Both of her parents were addicted to drugs and she was disappointed that they had not been sober during her visit. She left their home feeling hurt and dissatisfied, and angry that she didn't get to spend quality time with them as she had hoped.

As she drew, Elissa talked about the conflicting feelings she harbored toward her parents. In recent years, her mother has been in a serious car accident, her father had encountered legal troubles and both had been written off by most of their extended family. Elissa felt genuine concern as well as responsibility for their wellbeing, but also intense anger at them and a hopelessness that they would never change. I asked Elissa why she wanted to draw Olaf and whether he related to her parents at all. She replied that Olaf was a character who was loving and supportive to everyone he encountered, which represented how she felt she should be to her parents. She also reflected on an annual trip she had taken with her parents to Disney World as a child, noting that "there were some good times, too." Elissa shared that it was often difficult for her to reconcile her positive memories of her parents with the negative ones. She blamed her parents for the harm their addiction had inadvertently caused her, but also cherished the fond memories of their time together.

From a logotherapeutic perspective, it seemed that Olaf may have represented the warm and comforting aspects of her family, which she was able to recall even when her parents were at their worst. Olaf stood for the positive memories of her family—a symbol that helped Elissa find the meaning in her relationship with them. He reminded her of why she continued to visit, even though she often left disappointed. With this insight, the image was no longer out of place; instead, I recognized it as Elissa's attempt to comfort herself in response to her painful and unsatisfying visit home. I asked if her parents liked Olaf, too; and though she couldn't answer definitively, she added snowflakes around the character using a technique that her mother had shown her. This led to her sharing a memory of drawing snowflakes in the winter with her mother, which was a positive recollection that prompted laughter. The snowflakes, like Olaf, seemed juvenile on the surface; but the associated nostalgia was clearly a comfort that Elissa needed in order to find meaning in her tenuous relationship with her parents.

Elissa's father passed away from an overdose two years after that session. His death came at the beginning of the COVID-19 pandemic, creating added pain and challenges. Elissa has come to art therapy sporadically since his death and has used her time to reflect on her comforting memories of her father. These memories allow her to separate her father from his addiction. She can recognize his noetic dimension and recall the characteristics that she loved about him. Although there were aspects of his life that caused her pain, Elissa has found meaning in these positive memories of her father.

Resilience

Creativity and imagination are among the characteristics of people who are described as resilient (Worrall & Jerry, 2007). The art of the Holocaust offers evidence that resilience was cultivated in the camps and ghettos through the use of creativity. The artwork also served as a reminder to people of what they had already endured and of their capacity to continue fighting for survival. My art therapy clients often perceive their struggle in therapy as evidence of their capacity to survive. Tara (a pseudonym) was a client I saw upon her discharge from an eating disorder facility. We worked together as she reacclimatized to her life and tolerated the changes in her body. At the time, her mother was in remission from the cancer that had led to Tara's obsession with health and wellness, eventually manifesting in an eating disorder. Two years after our termination, Tara contacted me to return to art therapy. Her mother's cancer was no longer in remission and chemotherapy was proving ineffective.

Tara, now 15, described feeling overwhelmed and scared, so I asked her to draw that feeling. Using chalk pastels, she filled the paper with disconnected, abstract shapes in various colors. The resulting image looked like a puzzle that had been pulled apart, with the pieces in close proximity, but no longer connected. Tara explained that she felt as though she "fell apart every day," but later recognized that she always put herself back together.

After she completed the drawing, we talked about her mother's condition. Tara sensed that her mother had given up hope and had resigned herself to the fact that her cancer was terminal. Tara stated that she did not know if she could endure her mother's death and questioned her own ability to pick herself up yet again. I acknowledged the reality of her situation and agreed that losing her mother would be devastating. After sitting with that heaviness, I asked her to look at her artwork again and consider how she had been able to put herself back together in the past. We recounted various times that Tara had felt as though she was falling apart, as depicted in her drawing, and how she always managed to put herself back together. Using her drawing as a metaphor, Tara was reminded of her capacity for resilience.

Tara and I met at the beginning of the COVID-19 pandemic, before I began seeing clients virtually. She talked about feeling at peace, despite the chaos in the world. Aware that she and her family had already been through so much, Tara was confident that they could weather the pandemic. She noted how her response was oddly calm, especially compared to her peers at school. She drew a face resembling Jesus looking over a mountain range to depict the sense of calm she was experiencing (Figure 10.3). I couldn't ignore the similarities between this drawing and Zofia Stępień's *Prayer* (Figure 9.3). Both suggested a feeling of calm and peace, despite the chaotic circumstances each was drawn in. The religious figures that feature prominently in both images show the artists' ability to self-transcend through a dedication to their faith. In her drawing, Tara recognized her own capacity for resilience.

Hope

Noticing that her younger sister was also struggling in response to their mother's illness, Tara brought Leah (pseudonym) to one of our sessions prior to our termination. Tara was concerned that Leah felt detached from the rest of their family and thought that engaging in art therapy together would help Leah feel more connected. At age 12, Leah was not given as much information about her mother's condition as her older siblings. She felt confused and nervous about her mother's prognosis, and she worried that she couldn't rely on her parents or siblings to provide her the details

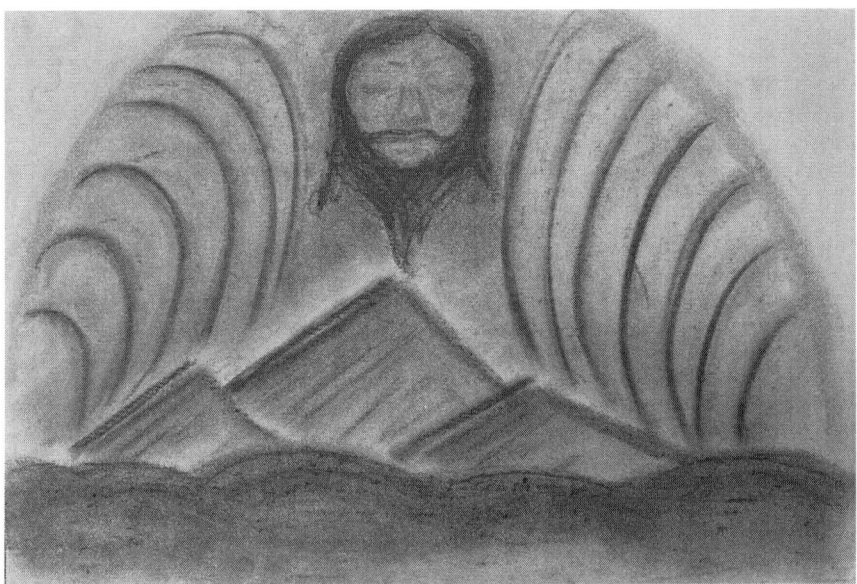

Figure 10.3 Calm, 2020. Chalk pastels on paper.

she wanted. Leah did know that plans for treatment were frequently changing and that her mother was often in immense pain. She stated that watching her family with the minimal information she had ultimately made her feel like a hopeless outsider.

I remembered my interview with Judy Godos-Jacobs, who had found a sense of hope through drawing butterflies and flowers in the Bergen-Belsen camp. In our conversion, she had recalled: "I think they were symbols of beautiful things you couldn't have in the camp. So, drawing them reminded the kids that they could have hope" (personal communication, 2017). Drawing images from her past had helped Godos-Jacobs access and define hope within her harsh and uncertain surroundings. The imagery reminded her that beauty could exist in the world and offered hope that she could one day experience it again. Depicting these symbols of hope reinforced Godos-Jacobs's hope in the future.

Because Leah felt lost and hopeless, I asked her to think of an image that had made her hopeful in the past. Leah responded that seeing the sun rise made her feel hopeful, and she began painting a memory from a recent camping trip: she recalled feeling full of hope and energy as she had watched the sunrise in the morning. This anecdote reminded me of Frankl's experiential value toward meaning, and I understood the sunrise as a reminder of Leah's capacity to find meaning. As she painted, Leah talked about how the sun was the one certainty in her life: it rose every morning and she always knew it was present, even if she couldn't see it behind the clouds. She used a range of colors to depict the sky, explaining that she could count on the sun to exist regardless of how the sky appeared. She experimented with clouding over the sun using other colors and seemed relieved when she could still see the image under the coats of paint.

As Leah painted, her affect changed. She considered how the assurance she felt in regard to the sun also pertained to her parents: though they weren't always transparent with her, she could count on them to be supportive and to answer her questions. Like the sun, their presence was consistent. Leah also began to recognize that if her mother did pass away, her impression on Leah would outlast her mortality. The relationship that she and her mother shared would always exist, even if her mother physically did not. The hopeful image of a sunrise reminded Leah of times she had felt hopeful in the past and she embraced the idea of hope once again.

At the time of writing, Leah and Tara's mother is in a stable condition. She participated in a clinical trial with positive results.

Connection

Art making allowed Holocaust victims to develop new and reinforce existing connections. Helga Hošková-Weissová and Thomas Geve both drew as a way to connect with the fathers from whom they had been separated. Artists working communally in camps and ghettos found a connection in creating together and for each other, as evidenced in the creative communities of Ravensbrück and Terezín. The desire for interpersonal connections can be viewed as an attempt to reconcile existential isolation (Yalom, 1980) and find meaning. Bruce Moon once told me that although the search for meaning is a solitary pursuit, meaning is found in the context of relationships. I thought about this recently in a session with Stacey (pseudonym), who recognized that creative writing was a connection she shared with her late grandmother.

Stacey is a 38-year-old single white professional, who has always enjoyed creative writing as a pastime. She initially came to art therapy for support with her poor body image, disordered eating and low self-esteem. In November 2021 she began a writing challenge, in which she wrote 50,000 words of a story that she had been workshopping for almost two decades. Stacey excitedly shared the updates she had made to her story in therapy each week, and I noticed how self-assured and confident she felt about her writing. Diving into this creative endeavor brought about a positive shift in Stacey's mood and confidence.

In December, when the challenge ended, Stacey reported feeling low. She continued writing, but noticed a drop in her mood and a reemergence of disordered behaviors that she had until recently been able to block. Stacey felt disappointed in herself and could not figure out why her affect had suddenly changed. In our session, she drew abstractly with chalk pastels—a favorite of hers—and tried to pinpoint what had triggered this change. While drawing, it occurred to Stacey that her late grandmother had always been encouraging of her writing and she felt disappointed that she could not share this accomplishment with her. She explained that writing was something that connected her to her grandmother and she grieved not being able to discuss her story together. Stacey had shared early iterations of her story with her grandmother and knew that she would have been proud to see its development. Upon further discussion, it became clear that although Stacey's grandmother had passed away five years prior, she was now recognizing the finality of her death.

I thought about how the creative act of writing had been a shared source of joy between Stacey and her grandmother. Like Hošková-Weissová's father, Stacey's grandmother encouraged her creative activity. As such, writing became more than a hobby; it was a symbol of the bond between them. Stacey explained that she felt proud of herself for committing herself to her writing, but grieved not being able to share that pride with the person who would have best understood. Stacey's low mood came from the grief she experienced in her grandmother's absence. She was relieved to have realized that insight, but the recognition brought back the pain she had felt when her grandmother passed away.

In our subsequent session, I asked Stacey if she wanted to continue exploring her relationship with her late grandmother. She began a collage using pictures from magazines that reminded her of how her grandmother had lived. She added pictures of flowers and talked about how her own love of gardening had been ignited by helping her grandmother in her garden. She glued down a picture of a baseball and talked about how her interest in the sport came from watching games with both of her grandparents. She added pictures of books to represent the hours she and her grandmother had read together, and the original writing she had always showed her grandmother. As Stacey compiled her collage, she realized that many of her interests and passions had grown out of her relationship with her grandmother. She seemed comforted by the awareness that she embodied so many of her grandmother's values. The connection was clearly deep, as the activities that Stacey found meaningful were all links to her grandmother. Writing had been a special bond between the two of them and Stacey felt a heavy sense of loss being unable to share her current writing with the person who had nurtured that passion. Collaging helped her to realize how significant an impact her grandmother had had on her, and she seemed comforted by the knowledge that she was carrying on her grandmother's legacies.

Concluding Thoughts

In each of the above cases, I was powerless to change the circumstances these clients had lived through. I could not erase Kelly's history of abuse; answer Allie's questions about her existence; deny the impact of Molly's disorder on her life; send Elissa's parents to rehab; find a cure for Tara and Leah's mother; or bring Stacey's grandmother back to life. What I could do was guide these clients to access the inner resources of their spiritual dimension. In doing so, each was able to find meaning in their painful situations, thus making the experience more bearable. The unyielding power of the human spirit is a function of one's capacity to access the spiritual dimension in an attempt to overcome adversity (Wong, 2009). By using this logotherapeutic approach, I provided my clients with an opportunity to activate their human potential.

I acknowledge the lack of diversity in the examples I have shared and wish that I could have drawn from a more heterogeneous group. I wanted to share authentic examples from my practice and, as I explained initially, my caseload lacks cultural diversity. I hope that art therapist readers are not dissuaded by this, but rather motivated to adopt the logotherapeutic attitude with a broader range of clients.

NON-CLINICAL EXAMPLES

Buddy

Although this chapter is based on how my clinical practice is informed both by my research and by logotherapy philosophy, I have noticed other examples of art being used as an opportunity to find meaning in other areas of my life. Since not all art therapists work in clinical settings, additional examples may serve to reinforce how one can find meaning through art making. The most salient example is that of my grandfather, who was known to all as Buddy. Although he was not a trained or professional artist, drawing and painting were prominent in Buddy's life. For years he attended a weekly oil painting class for senior citizens, where he painted portraits of almost everyone in our family. He moved on to Jewish imagery, followed by a series of Chagall's windows, and then back to portraits. He eventually added a portrait drawing class to his routine and briefly experimented with a clay class. He even painted mermaids on the bottom of the inground swimming pool in his backyard, which he touched up every year before opening the pool for summer.

Buddy constantly made art. He drew faces on his daily newspaper when talking on the phone and more faces on napkins while he waited for his food at a restaurant. He learned how to make origami and began folding napkins and papers after he had drawn on them. Art making seemed instinctual to him and he always supported my interest in art. He occasionally took me to classes with him and introduced me to oil painting at a young age. Some of the artwork that I included in my college application portfolio had been made when I was sitting next to him in a senior citizens' art class.

Early in his 90s, Buddy's physical health declined. When he was sent to a rehabilitation facility after a fall, I brought him a sketchbook and colored pencils. He drew every day, mostly portraits of other patients and staff. At one point, a patient asked Buddy if he would draw a portrait of her granddaughter. Another patient did the same and insisted on paying him for his work. Less than a year after he had been discharged, Buddy returned to the facility. The staff remembered him and one nurse admitted she was glad to see him back because she had wanted him to draw her portrait. He was modest about his drawings, but always happy to comply with what others requested.

He told me later that the drawing materials I brought were his saving grace: "What was I going to do—sit there and look at the walls?" Although he was bound to a wheelchair, his mind remained sharp. The idea of losing his cognitive abilities frightened him and he insinuated that drawing kept his mind active. I know that his drawing also helped him distinguish himself from other patients at the facility who were not as cognitively sound.

Buddy's health declined rapidly in February 2020. Once again, he was sent to a rehab facility; and once again, I brought pencils and paper. We drew together when I visited and I noticed evidence of cognitive decline in his work. I had been exposed to his drawings my entire life and the one he started during our visit was visibly different. I knew that he was coming to the end of his life and vowed to visit him every weekend. The following Saturday I tried to get him to draw again, but he struggled. He drew an outline of a head, but couldn't move on to other features. He kept tracing the outline of the head over and over, and seemed stuck and frustrated with himself. Portrait drawing had come so naturally to him and it pained me to see him unable to complete a task that had previously been effortless. He passed away the following week, aged 96.

Buddy lived a long and full life. I am reminded of him and his drawings when I reflect on the themes that arose in my interviews. Miriam Alon said that making art was like breathing to her mother Halina, and I would have said the same of Buddy. He found meaning in retirement by attending weekly art classes and connected to others by drawing their portraits. He studied faces and took in the distinctive features of his models. He found meaning in drawing at the rehab facility, noting that this hobby made his time there more tolerable. He chose how he would exist within the facility, and that was as an artist. Like Alfred Kantor, Buddy assumed the role of observer and felt he had a purpose greater than that of a patient. Art was something that always connected us and deepened the meaning in our relationship.

Brian's Dots

As I was concluding this text, I came across a pointillist artist whose story illustrates the meaning-finding potential of art. Brian Delozier grew up in Eastern Pennsylvania as an active kid and teenager, who described himself as "always in motion." His life-style changed abruptly after a skiing accident left him paralyzed at age 16. He held out hope that he would regain mobility and eventually learned to walk with crutches. Although doctors told him he was fortunate to have made any progress, Brian was devastated at the realization that he would never fully recover. With no sense of hope, he fell into a depression.

But one day, Brian decided to make a change. He realized, "I could go on like this indefinitely, and that was even scarier than trying to jump out and try something new" (personal communication, December 4, 2021); so he planned a trip to Hawaii to search for meaning. He was determined to find a new passion for life. He pushed himself to meet new people and eventually met an artist who suggested that he make art. Brian was skeptical: he had never been interested in art and did not even have full use of his hands. But the artist was persistent; and "one day, I picked up a marker and it felt comfortable to make dots. So I just started making dots." That moment was a turning point and soon Brian developed a passion for art. He developed a distinct technique in which he draws the outline of a picture on paper or canvas, then fills in the drawing one dot at a time. The result is a unique, colorful work of art. For the past 14 years, Brian has created hundreds of these drawings and exhibited across the United States. Toward the end of our conversation, Brian said:

> So I started making dots, and over the years, it has been more than just an outlet; it has changed my life. All this beauty comes from suffering. It transforms pain into beauty. It's never easy and I still struggle, but I always have art to transform what I'm going through (B. Delozier, personal communication, December 4, 2021).

Brian's tenacity is inspiring and his story perfectly highlights Frankl's philosophies. Brian demonstrated the will to meaning by deciding to find a way to live within his constraints. He recognized his responsibility to find meaning and did so by searching beyond what he knew of himself and his world. He discovered a love of art and committed himself to a career as an artist. He recognized that his suffering led him to find meaning in his art; and though he continues to suffer, he no longer feels despair. Through self-transcendence, Brian has found meaning through his art making.

CONCLUSIONS

Through these clinical and non-clinical examples, it is clear that art making can lead an individual to find meaning. This was also evident in the art of the Holocaust. Despite the inhumane conditions, individuals in Nazi camps and ghettos who made art were able to retain their humanity by engaging in a pursuit that, although dangerous, paradoxically strengthened them spiritually (Moreh-Rosenberg, 2016). Making art did not change the grotesque circumstances that those individuals endured.

Although their creativity supported a type of psychic survival (Moreh-Rosenberg, 2016), it did not ensure physical survival. In fact, some artists were brutally punished when their Nazi captors discovered their works (Green, 1978). What art making did offer was an opportunity to engage authentically by contemplating, exploring and ultimately sharing their lived experience. The artists assuaged their suffering by finding a meaning and purpose with their circumstance. That gave them the strength to continue fighting for survival. Art therapists and other clinicians cannot change the suffering our clients experience; it is beyond our capacity to make such significant changes. What we can do, however, is support our clients in finding a meaning which helps them to persevere through adversity. As was seen in the examples of artists creating in captivity, the art-making process can help an individual to access the distinctive resources of their spiritual dimension to find meaning.

Schneider (2015) asserted that psychotherapists can limit their capabilities if they focus primarily on "secondary conditions" (p. 23) such as poor emotion regulation, brain imbalances and irrational thoughts, and thereby neglect an exploration into deeper dimensions of existence. He argued that humankind's "precariousness as creatures" (p. 23) is the root of mental health concerns and therefore should be examined in therapy. The artists of the Holocaust engaged in this very type of deep self-exploration, showing that art has the power to lead an individual to deeply contemplate the meaning of their existence. By incorporating logotherapeutic philosophy into art therapy practice, I do not limit this work to psychiatric symptoms and causes, but rather invite clients to engage in an exploration that taps into their spiritual dimension. In this way, art therapists might consider this capacity of art to evoke the spiritual dimension and engage clients on an existential level.

I initiated a study of artwork from the Holocaust with the implicit feeling that it would reveal benefits that are connected to art therapy theories. In interviews with survivors, I learned that art making bolstered their sense of identity, hope, comfort, autonomy and resilience; affirmed their existence; strengthened interpersonal connections; and provided an opportunity to serve as a witness. These benefits contributed to a personal sense of meaning. Although their physical and psychological capacities were harmed, art making allowed their spiritual dimension to thrive. In recognition that these themes are inherent aspects of humanity, I have since structured my clinical work to help build these capacities within my clients. If, as Wong (2009) wrote, "the human spirit is the most important resource in psychotherapy, because it is the basis for recovery and resilience" (pp. 86–87), then art therapists and other practitioners can strive to develop and support the noetic aspect of their clients' existence. In doing so, we invite our clients to access their unique inner resources and take responsibility for healing.

REFERENCES

Amishai-Maisels, Z. (1993). *Depiction and interpretation: The influence of the Holocaust on visual arts.* Tarrytown, NY: Pergamon Press.

Costello, S. J. (2016). Towards a tri-dimensional model of happiness: A logo-philosophical perspective. In *Logotherapy and existential analysis.* Cham, Switzerland: Springer, pp. 343–363.

Frankl, V. (1959/2006). *Man's search for meaning* (5th ed.) (I. Lasch, trans.). Boston, MA: Beacon Press.

Frankl, V. (2004). *On the theory and therapy of mental disorders: An introduction to logotherapy and existential analysis* (J. Dubois, trans.). New York, NY: Routledge.

Frankl, V. E. (2014). *The will to meaning: Foundations and applications of logotherapy*. London, England: Penguin.

Graber, A. V. (2004). *Viktor Frankl's logotherapy: Method of choice in ecumenical pastoral psychology*. Lima, OH: Wyndham Hall Press.

Green, G. (1978). *The artists of Terezín*. New York, NY: Hawthorn Books.

Idinopulos, T. A. (1977). Humanistic education in an inhuman age. *CrossCurrents, 26*(4), 407–415.

Kapitan, L. (2009). The art of liberation: Carrying forward an artistic legacy for art therapy. *Art Therapy, 26*(4), 150–151. Doi: 10.1080/07421656.2009.10129618

Leclerc, J. (2011). Re-presenting trauma: The witness function in the art of the Holocaust. *Art Therapy, 28*(2), 82–89, doi: 10.1080/07421656.2011.580181

Leontiev, D. (2016). Logotherapy beyond psychotherapy: Dealing with the spiritual dimension. In *Logotherapy and Existential Analysis*. Cham, Switzerland: Springer pp. 277–290.

Makarova, E. (2001). *Friedl Dicker-Brandeis*. Los Angeles, CA: Tallfellow/Ever Picture Press.

Monnig, E. (2014). Coping strategies of Jewish children who suffered the Holocaust. *Arizona Journal of Interdisciplinary Studies, 3*, 42–57.

Moreh-Rosenberg, E. (2016). The art from the Holocaust. Cologne, Germany: Wienand Verlag.

Morris, F. J. & Willis-Rauch, M. (2014). Join the art club: Exploring social empowerment in art therapy. *Art Therapy, 31*(1), 28–36.

Overton, S. L. & Medina, S. L. (2008). The stigma of mental illness. *Journal of Counseling & Development, 86*(2), 143–151.

Reker, G. T. & Peacock, E. J. (1981). The life attitude profile (LAP): A multidimensional instrument for assessing attitudes toward life. *Canadian Journal of Behavioural Science/Revue Canadienne Des Sciences Du Comportement, 13*, 264–273. doi: 10.1037/h0081178

Rogina, J. M. (2015). Noogenic activation in the clinical practice of logotherapy and existential analysis (LTEA) to facilitate meaningful change. *The International Forum for Logotherapy, 38*, 1–7.

Rosenberg, P. (2009, March). Art during the Holocaust. *Jewish Women's Archive*. http://jwa.org/encyclopedia/article/art-during-holocaust.

Schulenberg, S. E., Hutzell, R. R., Nassif, C. & Rogina, J. M. (2008). Logotherapy for clinical practice. *Psychotherapy, 45*(4), 447–463. doi: 10.1037/a0014331

Schneider, K. (2015). The case for existential (spiritual) psychotherapy. *Journal of Contemporary Psychotherapy, 45*(1), 21–24. doi: 10.1007/s10879-014-9278-8

Sousa, D. (2015). Existential psychotherapy the genetic-phenomenological approach: Beyond a dichotomy between relating and skills. *Journal of Contemporary Psychotherapy, 45*(1), 69–77. doi: 10.1007/s10879-014-9283-y

Southwick, S. M., Lowthert, B. T. & Graber, A. V. (2016). Relevance and application of logotherapy to enhance resilience to stress and trauma. In *Logotherapy and existential analysis*. Cham, Switzerland: Springer, pp. 131–149.

Spenser, T. & Tarsi, A. (eds.) (2001). *Art and medicine in Ghetto Theresienstadt: Drawings from the years 1942–1944* [exhibition catalogue].

Wix, L. (2009). Aesthetic empathy in teaching art to children: The work of Friedl Dicker-Brandeis in Terezín. *Art Therapy, 26*(4), 152–158. doi: 10.1080/07421656.2009.10129612

Wong, P. T. (2009). Meaning therapy: An integrative and positive existential psychotherapy. *Journal of Contemporary Psychotherapy, 40*(2), 85–93. doi: 10.1007/s10879-009-9132-6

Wong, P. T. P. (2014). Viktor Frankl's meaning seeking model and positive psychology. In A. Batthyany & P. Russo Netzer (eds.). *Meaning in existential and positive psychology*. New York, NY: Springer

Worrall, L. & Jerry, P. (2007) Resiliency and its relationship to art therapy. *Canadian Art Therapy Association Journal, 20*(2), 35–53. doi: 10.1080/08322473.2007.11434772

Yalom, I. (1980). *Existential psychotherapy*. New York, NY: Basic Books.

EPILOGUE

I began this research in order to better understand the meaning and impact of Holocaust art and art creation. I was introduced to the phenomenon of Holocaust art around the same time that I was introduced to art therapy and the two have since been entwined in my mind. The opportunity to delve deeper into this subject has enabled me to better articulate how the art of the Holocaust has become such a critical component of my art therapy practice. I started my research journey by searching for qualitative commonalities between Holocaust art and art therapy, and found that both are examples of an outlet or expression and both relate to mastery and autonomy. While interesting points of comparison, these insights were surface level and based only on what I had read or surmised from the peripheral. In completing a phenomenological inquiry, I was able to access a more profound sense of the rationale behind Holocaust artwork and to recognize that the artists created to uphold the most human aspect of their existence.

In closing this text, I would like to return to the discussion in Chapter 1 of esthetic versus documentation. My conclusion was that the art of the Holocaust is meaningful in its service to both functions. The artwork made in captivity provides firsthand evidence of the horrors of the Holocaust, with similarities in content from artworks made in varying camps and ghettos corroborating the atrocities that occurred. These works document the daily struggle that victims faced not only to survive, but to retain their sense of personhood. What makes the artworks esthetically beautiful is the humanity that they embody in the face of inhuman oppression. Although many were created with improvised materials, the desire of the victim artists to create them represents the strength of the human spirit.

For some, however, it seems difficult to view small sketches on scraps of paper as art, when art is typically categorized as something grand and skillfully rendered, fit to hang on a wall. Indeed, although he did not delve into the abundance of artwork made by individuals in captivity, Viktor Frankl noted the absurdity of the concept of art made in a camp, asking: "Is there such a thing in concentration camps? It rather depends on what one chooses to call art" (2006, p. 41). This question of what to define as art has come up in both my research and my practice. Some survivors who I met with disregarded their artworks, and those of other captives, since they were made so primitively. These individuals were reluctant to consider such small, seemingly insignificant pieces as art, when they lacked traditional esthetic beauty.

This dismissive attitude toward amateur art also comes up in art therapy sessions. I have worked with clients who are hesitant to engage in the art-making process. They are adamant that if they are not talented or trained artists, their artwork cannot possibly be good and is therefore not worth making. I also see clients who minimize the significance of their artwork if it does not meet certain esthetic criteria. I strive to relieve my clients of this self-imposed burden and remind them that conventional beauty is not the goal of art making as a therapeutic practice—just as it was not the goal of art creators during the Holocaust. What I value as an art therapist is the expression of humanity that shines through in my clients' art. Their art is an opportunity to share a piece of them that is deeper than psychiatric symptoms.

The art-making process is a chance to find meaning in the midst of a bleak or challenging experience.

The ability to maintain a sense of humanity, regardless of external dehumanizing factors, is accentuated by the artists of the Holocaust. Although the artwork has been studied by other scholars as important evidence of visual culture from historical, cultural and art historical perspectives, it also evidences the persistence of human characteristics that are often witnessed by art therapists. The situation of the Holocaust is unique and unparalleled; however, the act of retaining human values in a dehumanizing situation through art is relevant to art therapists in myriad environments. Idinopulos (1977) stated that: "The great truth we have to learn from the Holocaust is how to keep the human spirit alive" (p. 408). The art of the Holocaust is an explicit example of the tenacity of the human spirit. I hope that art therapists reading this are reminded of art's ability to humanize individuals in even the most dehumanizing of situations. By engaging in art making, art therapists can guide clients to reclaim and bolster a potentially lost or faded sense of self.

INDEX

Page numbers in italics refer to figures. Page numbers in bold refer to tables.